DYNAMIC STRENGTH

DYNAMIC STRENGTH

BY HARRY WONG

UNIQUE PUBLICATIONS

DISCLAIMER

      Please note that the publisher of this instructional book is NOT RESPONSIBLE in any manner whatsoever for any injury which may occur by reading and/or following the instructions herein.

      It is essential that before following any of the activities, physical or otherwise, herein described, the reader or readers should first consult his or her physician for advice on whether or not the reader or readers should embark on the physical activity described herein. Since the physical activities described herein may be too sophisticated in nature, it is *essential that a physician be consulted.*

UNIQUE PUBLICATIONS INC., 1990
All rights reserved.
Printed in the United States of America.
ISBN: 0-86568-013-2
Library of Congress No.: 80-53545

 **UNIQUE PUBLICATIONS**
4201 Vanowen Place
Burbank, CA 91505

I dedicate this book to my late father, Nam Wong. He would always say,"Develop yourself, mentally first, physically second. Be unique and imaginative. Reach for the stars, for they will be yours, not his or mine." Thanks Dad... I didn't forget.

Contents

ACKNOWLEDGEMENTS

I would like to express my gratitude to my first and current teacher, Sifu Jimmy H. Woo of El Monte, California. As if he were a second father, his teachings have had a tremendous impact on my life. The qualities of respect, confidence outstanding character and an understanding of dynamic strength and the use of all the elements of the human body are just a fragment of the values for which I am indebted to him. He is truly a master of all, because he is a master of himself.

Sifu Daniel K. Lee is another teacher of the highest caliber. He unselfishly shares his vast knowledge of the many martial arts he has mastered, Tai Chi Chuan being his favorite. Understanding of the Yin and Yang, of strategy and the reality of combat, and of how to create and sharpen my tools are only a fraction of what he has taught me. I am honored and privileged to study under his humble guidance and fantastic ability.

Finally, without the encouragement and inspiration of Curtis F. Wong, publisher of Unique Publications, this book would just be an idea. Instead, it has materialized. I honor our many years of friendship and look forward to many more.

Also, sincere thanks to Sandra Segal, book editor, for her patience and long hours of hard work in preparing this book; to David M. King and Ed Ikuta for their expert knowledge in photography; to Mark Komuro and Alan Takemoto for their art direction.

Introduction

Why should anyone take up an exercise program like dynamic strength? In part, the answer is self-evident. Your physical well-being affects how you feel about yourself, how others react to you, and how well you're able to perform in every aspect of your life. If your body is strong and healthy, you will have a positive attitude and feel capable of surmounting any problems which arise in day to day life. On the other hand, if your body is weak and easily fatigued, you may feel powerless to reach your goals. A regular exercise program is the fastest way to make your body look and feel the way you want it to, to substitute strength and energy for flabbiness, weakness, and exhaustion. Persistence in following your program is the key to achieving these goals.

Dynamic strength is a unique exercise program, as it offers all the benefits of weight training without using weights. You will be able to strengthen your muscles, increase your power, and improve your physique without the common problems of weight training—strains, torn ligaments or tendons, back injuries, etc. You will also be able to avoid the weightlifter's problems of "cheating," that is, not moving the weight along the full range of motion from complete extension of a joint to complete contraction of a muscle. Cheating, often caused when a beginner uses too heavy weights, has improper instruction, or is simply lazy, leads to incomplete development of strenth and a loss of flexiblity. Because dynamic strength does not use weights, this problem can be completely avoided.

In dynamic strength, your muscles gain in strength by working against other muscles in your body, rather than against weights. You regulate the resistance in each exercise by changing the amount of tension with which you perform each exercise. The amount of tension will naturally increase as all your muscles become stronger. Dynamic strength has some similarities to isometirc type exercises in which muscles push or pull against each other. However, isometrics emphasize static exercises which stress only a single point of the range of movement or flexibility. In dynamic tension, all exercises are performed with a full range of movement. The resistance which develops the muscles is *dynamic*, thus enhancing the muscle's range of flexibility, speed and power in motion.

It may be difficult to understand how you can build muscles without using weights. Try this simple exercise: Imagine you are holding a barbell in front of you. Feel the weight of it in both hands. Now slowly raise the imaginary weight, feeling its resistance as you lift it up. Note that your biceps tense as if you were really lifting the weight. If you do the exercise very slowly with a great deal of tension, you will begin to build bulk. If you do more repetitions with less tension, you will increase the definition of the muscle.

Dynamic strength imparts a body awareness which is vital for the martial arts. By becoming aware of each individual muscle and separately increasing its strength, you will gain more control in your power. Your balance, grace and flexibility will increase. You will be able to focus your strength to achieve your aims, using no more nor less than is required. You will have made your power a part of yourself.

As you review the warm-ups and dynamic strength exercises that follow, you will note that many include martial arts stances and have specific application to martial arts techniques. These applications will be clearly described and demonstrated with each pertinent exercise.

In the dynamic strength exercise program, the mind becomes stronger and more capable as the body strengthens. Dynamic strength begins by focusing your mind and gaining awareness of your various sensory perceptions: touch (feeling); sight (not only vision, but the sense of being alert); smell (breathing); hearing (listening); and taste. All of these elements are coordinated and brought into focus during dynamic strength exercises. This requires tremendous concentration. However, once mastered, your control will be physically and mentally enhanced. You should strive for concentration coordinated with relaxation.

The first section of this book explains the mental aspect of dynamic strength. This chapter may be the most vital one in the book. Without proper mental preparation in your exercise program, you will not be able to obtain its full effect. With a positive mental attitude, you will be successful in achieving your goals not only in your physical development but also in many other areas of your life.

The second section of this book covers the warm-up exercises which should be performed before beginning each exercise session. The dynamic strength execises are then covered thoroughly in the third section with photos and complete explanations of the steps involved. A training schedule which is flexible enough to fit anyone's goals follows.

Preliminaries: Mental Preparation and Breathing

Attitude

Attitude, rather than aptitude, is the chief ingredient for success. Before you begin this exercise program, stop and decide exactly what your goals are. Do you want powerful muscles? Better health? Greater speed? Increased skills in the martial arts? Having a clear idea of what you want to achieve is the first step towards reaching your goal.

Now that you have decided what you are aiming for, you must consider how determined you are to reach your goals. The degree of achievement that you will be able to attain is limited only by the magnitude of the goal you set for yourself and by the desire you have to achieve it. By thinking positively, you can create the mental, emotional, and physical environment most suited for reaching your goal. You must visualize what you want to happen and convince yourself that you are capable of it. With this attitude, you will have the will power and confidence to remake yourself.

It is vital to have this positive attitude each time you begin your exercises. Confidence is the main ingredient for a successful positive attitude. When starting an exercise series, never think, "Oh, I can't do that." That thought alone may prevent you from making any further gains. Instead, use your mind to progress faster by imagining yourself effortlessly doing the exercises and quickly strengthening your body. In this way, you will learn how to harness your mind's energy, and discipline it to eliminate negative, weakening thoughts. Your control of your mind in this situation will extend to other situations. By learning to control yourself, you will eventually be able to control others.

The power of the mind can change your old unhealthful habits to new habits. Changing your habits must be done in order to grow. For example, if you try to develop the habit of holding your stomach in and standing up straight, a correct posture will eventually become natural to you. You will then have the double benefit of learning you have the ability to change yourself and of incorporating a habit that will make you look better and have better feelings about yourself.

Approach each exercise session with enthusiasm, and consider it an opportunity to approach yourself with respect and confidence, to give your muscles the workout which they require, and to improve yourself. You should take your exercise program seriously, as it may be the most important thing you do for yourself each day. Remember that you have put aside this time for concentrating on your own person.

Your exercise session should not be a chore. If you find yourself approaching an exercise session with a negative feeling, do not begin to exercise. Either go on to some other activity and begin your exercises when you can do them with a positive spirit, or sit quietly for a few minutes, thinking about your goals and about the good feelings you get from exercising your muscles. If you force yourself to exercise, you will not do the exercises in the right spirit and you will not fully benefit from them.

Concentration and Awareness

By freeing your mind of any negative thoughts, you will be able to enhance your self-awareness and concentration. Focusing your mind on your physical being is one of the most essential parts of your exercise session.

Most people go through life completely oblivious to the way their bodies feel. They become aware of their bodies only when experiencing pain through cramping, stiffness, etc. Take the first step towards self-awareness now, as you are reading this book. Think about and listen to your body. Do your neck and shoulders feel stiff? Are you in an uncomfortable position? Are you completely relaxed? If any parts of your body feel tense, begin to consciously relax them now.

Body awareness is essential when you are engaged in your exercises. When preparing for an exercise session, first stand up straight and become aware of how each part of your body feels. Locate any areas of tension or stiffness, and concentrate on relaxing them as you have just done. You should feel relaxed, but do not become drowsy or allow your muscles to become heavy.

When practicing each exercise, try to be deeply aware of the experience of the exercise. How does your entire body feel? How do the individual muscles involved react? Are you experiencing any pain or stress?

After practicing each exercise several times, you will begin to realize when you are doing an exercise exactly right. All of your muscles will coordinate perfectly and you will experience the right amount of tension. When you get this feeling of rightness, concentrate on locking it into your body and mind. Tune in to your senses and try to remember every aspect of your feeling so that you can achieve the same sensations each time you repeat the exercise. Concentrate on achieving and maintaining that feeling as you exercise in a comfortable rhythm. With each repetition, you should also attempt to discover new sensations which will contribute to perfecting your performance. Continually remind yourself of exactly what you are trying to achieve with each particular exercise.

To enhance the effects of the exercises, focus on the part of the body for which the exercise is intended. When you are doing curls, for example, concentrate on the muscles in your wrists, forearms, biceps and shoulders. Visualize them working and growing stronger. When doing flexibility exercises, focus on the muscles, ligaments, and tendons stretching and elongating and becoming more flexible. Be wary of performing your exercises simply by rote. Instead of performing like a mindless robot only on a physical plane, use your mind to control specific muscles, commanding them to perform and respond in the desired manner. Always attempt to unify your mind's consciousness with your body's actions.

If you can, watch yourself in a full length mirror while doing the exercises. This will help prevent you from doing them incorrectly because of habitual poor body posture. You will be able to see how your whole body is involved in each exercise, and you will start to isolate the different muscles and muscle groups involved. You will also be able to see improvements in your physique, which will be a helpful motivating factor in continuing your program.

Eventually, you will be separately aware of every muscle and muscle group in your body, and be able to flex muscles that other people may not even know they have. This knowledge of how your body works will give you tremendous control in creating the physical self you desire.

Equilibrium and Harmony

By exercising with a focused awareness of your body, your mental and physical selves will begin to work in harmony, and join in a state of relaxed alertness. Because of the problems that arise in daily life, your mind may be sending messages to your body to become tense. Your shoulders, arms, and back may begin to ache. By exercising and learning to listen to your body, you will both discharge the tension and learn to relax your muscles. It will become easier and easier for your mind to tell your body to relax, until this relaxed alertness becomes your natural state of being. Conflicts within your inner being will be considerably reduced, thus enabling you to be more efficient and effective not only in dynamic strength exercises but in your daily life as well. You will gain a psychological and physiological equilibrium that will extend throughout your life.

Breathing

Breathing is one of the most overlooked functions of the human body. We take air for granted, probably because breathing is an innate process, and we don't have to purchase air like food or water. Without air, the human body cannot survive beyond a few minutes.

The Chinese term for air is *chi*, and it is commonly referred to as the life force. Chi is best described as an intrinsic energy stored and nurtured in an area three inches below the navel. This area is called the *tan tien*. By breathing low or abdominally, your chi will sink down to the tan tien. Controlled, concentrated breathing directed by the mind results in chi circulation throughout the body. The rotation exercises help unblock all the passages in the spine, waist, elbows, wrists, knees and ankles so chi can circulate without interruption. One's goal should be to have the ability to harness the energy created by chi and use the mind to direct and flow it anywhere internally or externally.

Proper breathing should be coordinated with all movements, relaxing the body by calming the mind. In order to motivate the chi to flow, breathing should be long and deep, slow and even.

In doing the exercises, inhale through your nose when you extend your arms upwards and outward, and exhale through your nose as you contract your arms or bring them downward. Since inhaling and exhaling are done through the nose, the mouth should be closed, with the tongue curled against the roof of the palate. The tongue should stick to the palate to insure that the salivary glands work continuously. The saliva should be swallowed to wet the throat, which aids in digestion. This method helps you concentrate on the chi sinking to the desired areas of development. Remember, proper breathing is essential to these exercises; inadequate respiration will retard your development.

Basic Warm-Ups

After you have prepared yourself mentally for dynamic strength, you must next prepare yourself physically with a series of warm-up exercises. These exercises stretch and stimulate all of the major muscle groups of the body. They loosen the joints, increase blood circulation, and awaken the body for more vigorous exercises.

Be sure to allow yourself plenty of time to do these exercises. Injuries may result if your body is not fully warmed up. Also, if your warm-up is incomplete, you will be less able to get the full benefit of dynamic strength. Everyone requires more or less time for warm-up preparation, depending upon your physical and mental condition. Let your body tell you when you've warmed up enough to begin the dynamic strength exercises. Remember to enjoy your warm-up sessions.

Before doing these exercises, review the chapter on mental preparation. Then, when you begin the warm-ups, concentrate on the parts of your body being affected. Think about and feel the stretching and elongating effects on the muscles, tendons, and ligaments and the loosening, lubricating effect the exercises have on your joints. Also visualize how the exercises are stimulating and strengthening your digestive system and your circulatory system. By concentrating, these exercises will have a beneficial effect on your internal organs as well as your limbs and muscles.

These warm-up exercises were developed in the tradition of the Shaolin monastery, the cradle of the martial arts. Legend has it that a holy monk, Bodhidharma, left his monastery in India to spread the Buddhist faith in China. After crossing the Himalayan Mountains, he entered the Shaolin monastery in the Shao Shih mountains. His first disciples, however, were too weak to stay awake during the lengthy meditation sessions. So Bodhidharma designed a series of exercises to strengthen his disciples' bodies and spirit. After engaging in these exercises daily, his students found that their bodies became strong and properly conditioned for the rigors of their spiritual path. Ultimately, these exercises were developed into a system of self-defense, which many believe is the basis of all kung-fu.

A multitude of different exercises have been developed. This book uses the common, popular ones most people are familiar with. However, many of them have been especially adapted to be more pertinent to the martial arts.

In order to gain the maximum benefits achievable with these exercises, you must approach them with an openness of mind, a positive spirit and an awareness of what your goals are.

Do the following before beginning your training session:

1. Stand in front of a mirror, feet shoulder width apart, and relax. Discard all negative thoughts.
2. Examine yourself in the mirror for a few minutes. Take inventory of yourself. Think about what you see and what you want to see.
3. Ask yourself how and what you feel.
4. Begin calming yourself by feeling that you are rooted to the ground by your feet.
5. Visualize and relax all your muscles. Imagine all your muscles hanging from a skeletal spine. Your facial muscles should also hang relaxed, but you should remain alert.
6. Listen to your body. Empty your mind of all thoughts.

CORE WARM-UP EXERCISES

The following seven exercises are the core of dynamic strength training. If you do no other exercises but these, you will still profit from this program. They provide a complete loosening and toning of your body, and prepare you for any exercises or athletic activities in which you participate.

NECK ROTATION

Since the neck joint is a pivot joint which allows a high degree of movement, the neck muscles have a 180 degree range of motion and can move the head to various angles. Because of this large range of motion, the neck particularly benefits from rotation exercises. Strong neck muscles also help protect your spinal cord from injury when the head is jerked, as in taking a blow.

DESCRIPTION

Stand erect with your feet together. Keep your legs straight, but do not lock your knees. Be sure your entire body, including your facial muscles, is relaxed. In every warm-up and dynamic strength exercise it it vital that you relax all parts of your body which are not being exercised. By doing this, you will be able to concentrate on the feelings you are getting in the muscles being exercised. Tuning into what your body is doing during each exercise is a vital part of dynamic strength.

Begin with your head erect, looking straight ahead. Then let your chin drop to your chest. Rotate your head back over your left shoulder, keeping the neck stretched to the side as far as it will go. Continue the rolling motion until you are looking at the ceiling. Then roll over your right shoulder, and finally, return your chin to your chest. Be sure to keep your shoulders in a relaxed position and avoid any bunching up which may occur. You should feel a gentle stretch, and you may hear a popping, grating sound in your neck. This is the sound of calcium deposits being broken up as you exercise. Eventually, your neck will roll smoothly and silently. Now reverse the motion and roll back the other way.

NUMBER OF REPETITIONS

Beginner: 12 rotations clockwise; 12 rotations counterclockwise
Intermediate: 24 rotations in each direction
Advanced: 36 rotations in each direction

COUNT

This exercise should be done to a count of 5.

1. chin against chest
2. head resting on left shoulder
3. head looking straight up at the ceiling
4. head resting on right shoulder
5. head again resting on chest

EFFECTS

This exercise will loosen and lubricate the neck joint and strengthen all of the neck muscles. The upper back muscles will also be stretched. After you have completed the exercise, try moving your head back and forth. It should feel looser and more flexible. The bands of muscles in your neck should feel relaxed and stretched.

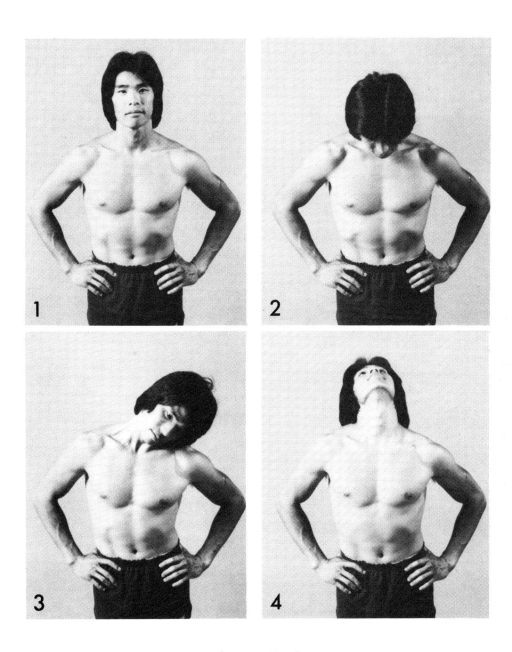

1. Stand erect with your feet shoulder distance apart.
2. Let your chin drop to your chest.
3. Rotate your head back over your left shoulder, keeping the neck stretched to the side as far as it will go.
4. Continue the rolling motion until you are looking at the ceiling.

NECK ROTATION

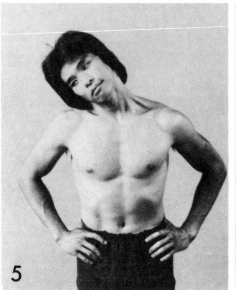 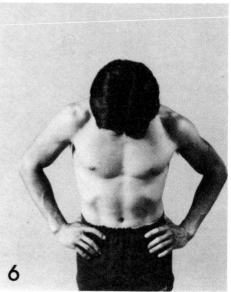

5. Roll over your right shoulder.
6. Return your chin to your chest.

UPPER TORSO ROTATION

The upper torso includes the shoulder joint and muscles, and all of the muscles of the upper back (trapezius or traps), lower back (latissimus dorsi or lats), upper chest and lower chest (pectoral muscles or pecs) and abdomen. The spinal cord also needs gentle stretching exercises to retain its flexibility and to prevent it from constricting and shrinking.

DESCRIPTION:

Stand erect with feet together, knees slightly bent. Lock your hips so they provide a stable base for the exercise. Put both hands behind the small of your back with palms facing down on the middle back. Your hands should be as high under your rib cage as possible. Using your hips as a base and your hands for support, bend your torso forward as far as it will go. Then, with a rotating move, swing to your left side. Continue the swing towards the back. When your torso is straight back, your head should still be looking forward, not up at the ceiling. Continue the rotation over your right side until you are back in the starting position. Then reverse the movement and rotate in the other direction.

As you do this exercise, you may feel a popping and cracking in your spine. This is just the normal sound of vertebrae loosening and tendons and ligaments adjusting to the unaccustomed movement.

NUMBER OF REPETITIONS

Beginner: 12 rotations clockwise; 12 counterclockwise
Intermediate: 24 rotations in each direction
Advanced: 36 rotations in each direction

COUNT

This exercise should be done to a count of 5.

1. rotation forward
2. left side
3. back
4. right side
5. center

EFFECTS

This is an excellent upper-body stretcher for the chest, waist, hips, and lower back muscles. It also loosens the spine, counteracting the stiffening of vertebrae which occurs with age and disuse. If your opponent aims or lands a punch on your upper body, you will be able to smoothly rotate your torso to evade the punch without losing your balance or yielding ground. As in all rotations, flexibility and strength will be enhanced.

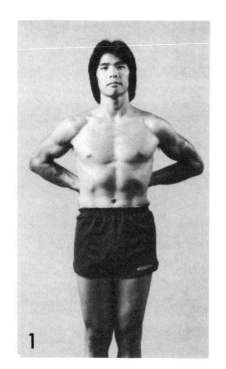

1

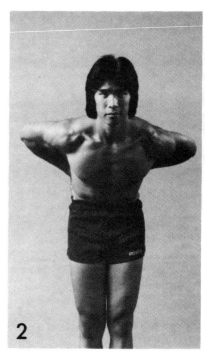

2

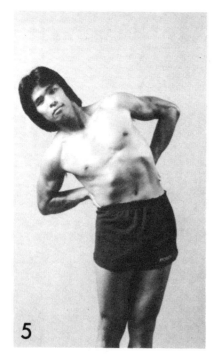

5

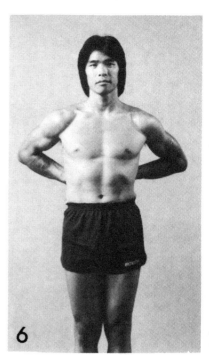

6

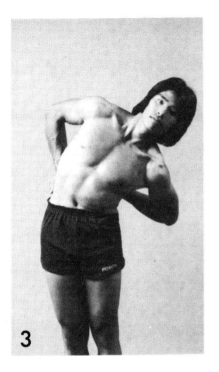

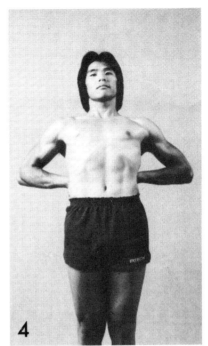

1. Stand erect with feet shoulder width apart. Both hands are palm down on the middle back.
2. Bend your torso forward as far as it will go.
3. With a rotating motion, swing to your left side.
4. Continue the swing towards the back.
5. Then rotate over the right side.
6. Return to the starting position.

SHOULDER ROTATION

Like the hip, the shoulder is a ball and socket joint which must be moved through its extreme range of motion to remain flexible. This joint is often neglected by athletes, sometimes to such an extent that they have trouble reaching behind them. In extreme cases, the shoulder joint can even "freeze," allowing only very limited motions.

DESCRIPTION

Stand in a bow and arrow stance. This stance, used in many exercises, is an erect stance, with feet at shoulder width. Shift your weight by turning your left foot out at a 45 degree angle. Bend your left knee, and move your right leg straight out, as far as you can, placing the right heel down first, lightly. There should be no weight on your right foot, so that you maintain the ability to lift it up. Then transfer your weight to the right lead foot by dropping its sole and pushing off from the left foot to the right. Your weight should now be seventy percent on the right leg and thirty percent on the rear leg. Both knees are slightly bent.

Standing in this bow and arrow stance, put your right hand down by your knees, palm parallel to the ground, as if resting on an imaginary stool. Your left arm should hang straight down at your side. Gently swing your left arm backwards, up and forward, making a complete circle. Your arm should be fully extended at all times.

Be sure your arm doesn't begin making a circle further away from your body. The circle made by your arm should be in as straight a line as possible close to your body.

On the backwards swing of the rotation, your hand will shift its position and gradually turn towards the back wall. At the height of the backwards swing, your palm should be in line with the back of your head.

On the forward movement of the rotation, your hand should slice through the air. Your hand should be straight as for a knife chop, with the palm facing in, parallel to the body. This stroke is much like an overhand swimming stroke.

Now take a bow and arrow stance with the left leg forward, and repeat the same rotation with the other arm. Your left hand will be resting on the imaginary stool. Begin swinging your right arm back, and go through the full cycle of rotations.

NUMBER OF REPETITIONS
Beginner: 12 rotations in each direction
Intermediate: 24 rotations in each direction
Advanced: 36 rotations in each direction

COUNT

This exercise should be done to a count which equals the number of rotations, i.e. one count for each rotation.

EFFECTS

This exercise loosens and lubricates the joint capsule in the shoulder. It also strengthens the shoulder muscle, all the muscles around the shoulder blade, the lower back, and the upper back muscles.

Increased flexibility and strength in your shoulder will help promote effective shoulder blocks. Instead of blocking a blow to the head with your whole body or by an arm movement, you will now be able to simply bring up your flexible shoulder. Your ability to escape from shoulder locks will also be improved. This exercise also increases the speed and extension of your arm movements.

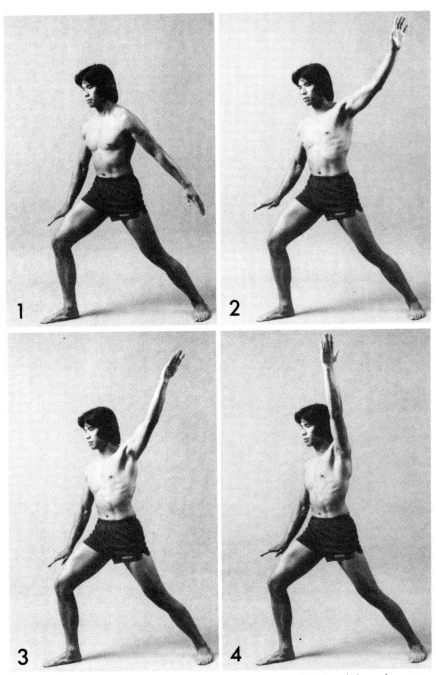

1. Standing in a bow and arrow stance, put your right hand down by your knees, palm parallel to the ground. Your left arm is hanging straight down at your side; then begin gently swinging your arm backwards.

2. As you swing back, your palm begins to face the back wall.

3. When you reach the extreme point of your backwards swing, reverse your hand so it now slices through the air.

4. Begin swinging the arm forward.

SHOULDER ROTATION

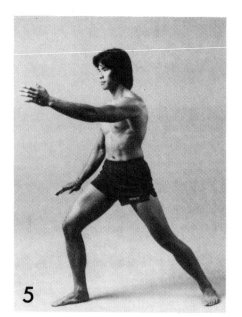 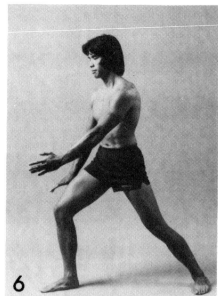

5. As you swing your arm down, be sure to keep your hips facing forwards.
6. Continue the downwards swing until your left arm returns to its original position.

ELBOW ROTATION

The elbow is a fairly delicate hinge joint which needs continual exercise to remain supple. The joint must be lubricated, and the muscles around the elbow joint in the forearm and in the upper arm need strength. Without the full range of motion in the elbow, blocks, punches, and any other arm movements will lack the necessary fluidity.

DESCRIPTION

Stand in a horse stance. The horse stance, used in many exercises in this book, is a relaxed stance with feet slightly beyond shoulder width (approximately four feet apart) with knees slightly bent.

Raise your right hand to the center line of your body (the line bisecting the body) with fingers pointing up. Position your left arm at the side of the body with elbow bent and palm up. Keeping your elbow stationary, rotate your right forearm counterclockwise until your palm is facing down. Next, rotate the forearm clockwise until it has returned to its original position. Then extend your right arm straight out in a finger jab. Finally, let your elbow sink until your arm has returned to its original position. Repeat with the left arm.

NUMBER OF REPETITIONS

Beginner: 8 rotations clockwise; 8 rotations counterclockwise
Intermediate: 16 rotations in each direction
Advanced: 24 rotations in each direction

COUNT

This exercise should be done to a count of 5.

1. palm down
2. palm up
3. finger jab
4. palm up
5. return to starting position

EFFECTS

By increasing flexibility in your elbow, this exercise helps you to raise your forearm from the elbow in one swift motion. This is invaluable in palm blocks. Instead of moving the entire arm, you will be able to bring up your forearm for a quick, subtle block.

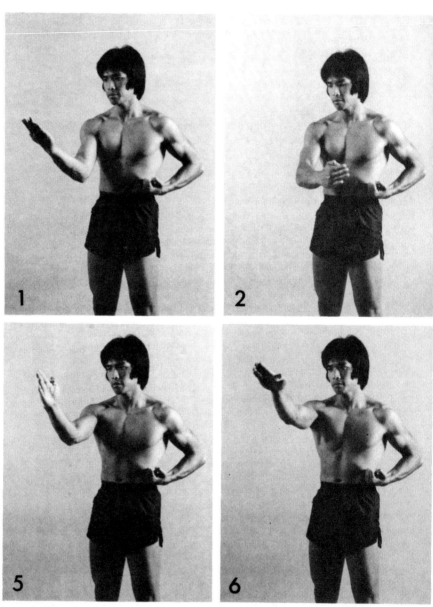

1. Standing in a horse stance, raise your right hand to the center line of the body, with fingers pointing up.
2. Keep the elbow stationary while you rotate your forearm counter-clockwise.
3. Continue rotating the forearm until your palm faces down.

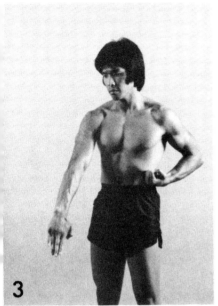

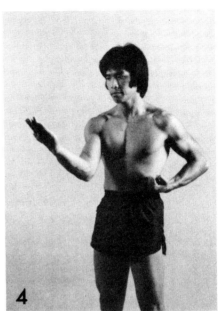

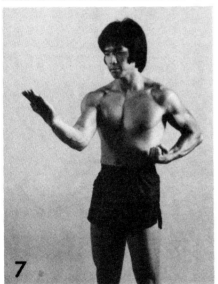

4. Then rotate your forearm clockwise until it has returned to its original position.

5. Begin turning your hand sideways...

6. And then extend it straight out in a finger jab.

7. Return your hand to the original position.

WRIST/FINGER STRETCHER

In a punch, the force of the entire body must pass through the wrist. A freely pivoting wrist joint and strong forearm muscles are necessary in any quick hand exchange for free flowing energy.

VARIATION: INNER STRETCH
DESCRIPTION

Begin in a horse stance. Position your elbow with your right arm in front of you and your hand palm up, forearm parallel to the body. Firmly hold the wrist with your left hand. Your left hand's fingers will hold the front of the right wrist, and your thumb will be behind the back of the right hand between the middle and ring fingers. Slowly lower your right forearm and hand, holding the wrist firmly with your left hand, and pressing gently with your thumb. Continue the sinking and pressing movements until your hand makes a 90 degree or slightly more acute angle with your wrist. Hold for ten seconds and then slowly come up.

VARIATION: OUTER STRETCH
DESCRIPTION

Begin in a horse stance. Position your right arm in front of you, elbow bent, palm down, forearm parallel to your body. Hold the back of the right hand with your left hand. Lower your right hand while pressing down with your left hand. Continue the sinking and pushing motion until your hand forms a 90 degree angle with the wrist. Hold for ten seconds. As you slowly come back up, raise the forearm only while maintaining the downward push of the left hand.

NUMBER OF REPETITIONS

Repeat five times with each hand

COUNT

In this exercise, hold at the point of tension for a count of ten in each of the positions.

EFFECTS

These exercises will give you a freely pivoting wrist joint, and strengthen the forearm muscles. You will also stretch the muscles of the hands and fingers. The loosening of the wrist is especially helpful in evading wrist locks. If your wrist is not flexible, the pain of having the wrist locked under pressure will disrupt your reactions. With this exercise, your wrists will have the flexibility to escape from the lock.

1. Stand erect, feet shoulder width apart. Use the fingers of your left hand to hold the front of your right wrist, and put your left thumb behind the back of the right hand.
2. Slowly lower your right forearm and hand, pressing gently with your your left thumb, until your hand makes a 90 degree angle with your wrist.
3. A side view of this exercise shows the tension in the arm and forearm.
4. The tension increases as the arm is pressed down.

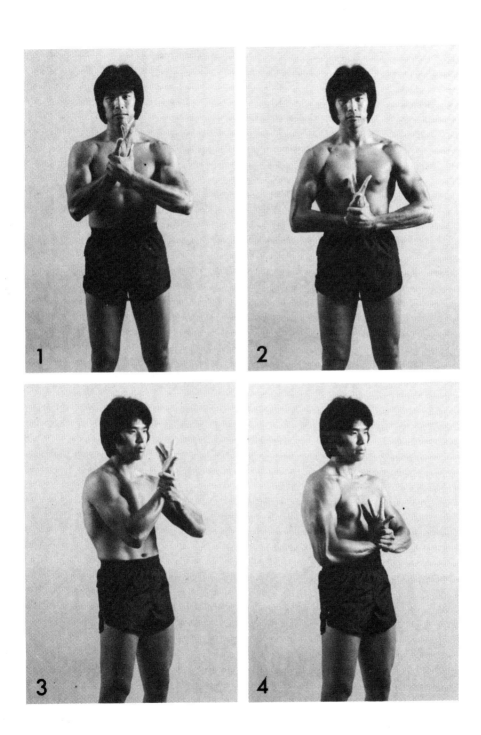

WRIST/FINGER STRETCHER

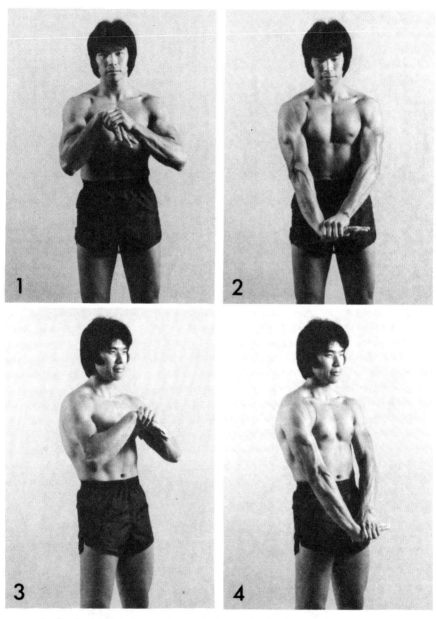

1. Beginning in a horse stance, hold the back of your right hand with the fingers of your left hand.
2. Lower your right hand while pressing down with your left hand until your hand forms a 90 degree angle with the wrist.
3. In this side view of the variation, note how both arms remain close to the body throughout the exercise.
4. Be sure to hold this position for a count of ten.

HIP ROTATION

The hip joint is a ball and socket joint which should have a smooth swiveling motion. Since ball and socket joints permit the greatest range of motion possible in the body, they must receive the fullest degree of exercise.

DESCRIPTION

Begin in a full horse stance. Put your hands behind you with your palms on your lower back. Keep your head as centered as possible. Supporting yourself with your hands, begin a pelvic thrust forward. Then in a circular movement, swing your hips to the left. Continue moving your hips through a complete circle. When you have returned to center position, reverse direction. You will feel the joints of the legs rotating in their pelvic sockets.

NUMBER OF REPETITIONS

Beginner: 12 rotations clockwise; 12 rotations counterclockwise
Intermediate: 24 rotations in each direction
Advanced: 36 rotations in each direction

COUNT

This exercise should be done to a count of 5.

1. forward
2. left
3. back
4. right
5. center

VARIATION

Instead of standing in a horse stance, stand with feet together, knees slightly bent. Rotate your pelvic area in a complete circle. You will probably not be able to make as large a circle in this position.

EFFECTS

This exercise will loosen up your pelvic area, hips, waist, lower back, spine, and the point where the legs join the hips. This increased flexibility helps in improving body balance, posture, and in strengthening your lower back and abdominal muscles. The pivoting of the hips will increase the power of your kicks. In offense and in defense, the transferring of weight from lead foot to rear foot neutralizes your opponent's attack.

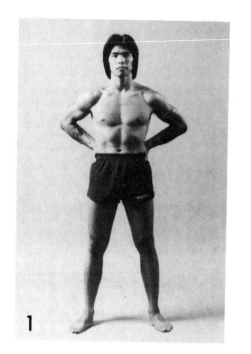

1

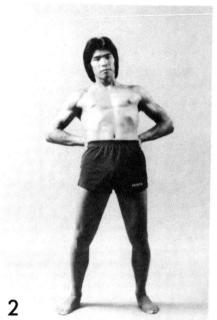

2

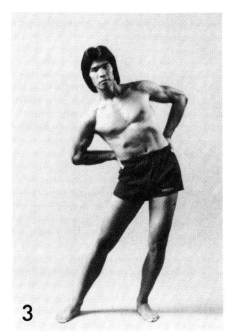
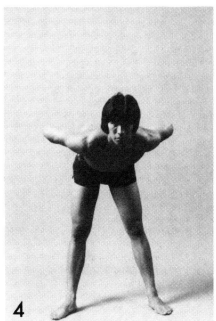

1. Begin with feet shoulder width apart, with your hands behind you, palms on your lower back.
2. Thrust your pelvis forward.
3. Swing your hips to the left in a circular movement.
4. Continue your circular movement to the back.
5. Then swing your hips to the right, and return to center.

KNEE ROTATION

The knee is a hinge joint which must bear almost the entire weight of your body. When you are sparring, it must endure fast starts and stops and wrenching twists which can injure this sensitive joint if it has not been conditioned by exercise.

DESCRIPTION

Stand with feet together, knees slightly bent. Place your hands on your knee caps. You should not apply any pressure, but merely feel the movement of the knees. Keeping the knees bent throughout the exercise, rotate the knees to the left. Continuing the circular movement, rotate them back, then right, and then return to the front. Reverse the motion and rotate in the other direction.

NUMBER OF REPETITIONS

Beginner: 8 rotations clockwise; 8 rotations counterclockwise
Intermediate: 16 rotations in each direction
Advanced: 24 rotations in each direction

COUNT

This exercise should be done to a count of 5 or more. It is important not to rotate so fast that a strain is put on the knees.

1. forward
2. left side
3. backward
4. right side
5. center

EFFECTS

This exercise helps lubricate and exercise the joint capsule of the knee, and strengthens the surrounding muscles to prevent injuries. The ankles also increase in flexibility, and the calves undergo a gentle stretch. This exercise will help enhance the speed and power of your kicks.

1. Stand erect, feet together, hands at your side.

2. Bend your knees and gently place your hands on your kneecaps.

3. Keeping your knees bent, rotate to the left.

4. Continue the circular motion backwards, then to the right.

Finally return to the original position.

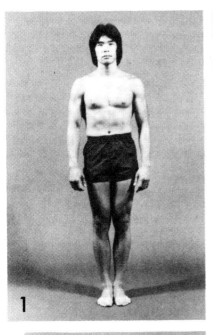

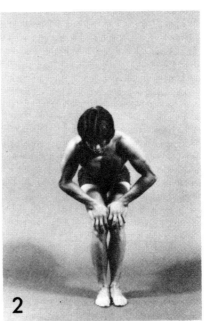

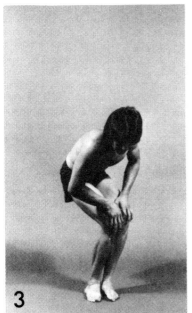

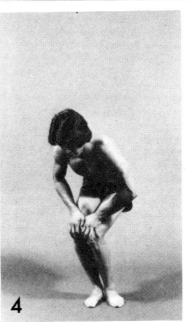

1

2

3

4

KNEE SWING

DESCRIPTION

Stand erect with legs at shoulder distance. Place your hands on your hips. Shift your weight onto your left foot. Your left knee should be slightly bent with your foot turned 45 degrees to the left. Raise your right leg, positioning your knee with your thigh parallel to the ground. Allow the calf to swing freely. Begin the rotation by swinging your lower leg straight out, and then begin a circular movement to the right. Repeat with your left leg. If you lose your balance, stop and relax all of your muscles. Feel the pull of gravity rooting and sinking you to the ground.

NUMBER OF REPETITIONS

Beginner: 12 rotations clockwise; 12 rotations counterclockwise with each leg
Intermediate: 24 rotations in each direction with each leg
Advanced: 36 rotations in each direction with each leg

COUNT

This exercise should be done in a single fluid motion, using a count of two.

EFFECTS

In addition to exercising the knee joint and the surrounding muscles, this exercise is particularly important in helping you develop balance through your awareness of relaxation and sense of sinking with the pull of gravity.

1. Stand erect, with legs shoulder width apart.
2. Shift your weight onto your left foot, and raise your right leg until your thigh is parallel to the ground.
3. Begin swinging your leg clockwise.
4. Continue the rotation until you return to the original position.

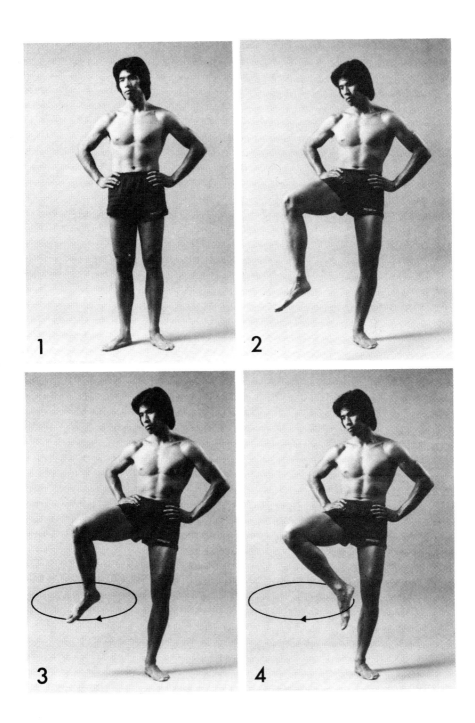

SUPPLEMENTARY WARM-UPS

These warm-ups supplement the core warm-up series, and should be done when you have the time. Each exercise provides excellent conditioning and stretching of different body areas. If you feel you have a weakness in any area, you may wish to concentrate on one of these exercises in addition to the core exercises. Add those exercises that you feel are compatible with your own specific wants and needs.

SHOULDER ROLL

Because the shoulder has a tremendous range of motion, it is valuable to use a variety of exercises to loosen it. Each exercise affects the joints and muscles in a slightly different way, providing a more comprehensive stretch. As these exercises also help you reduce tension in your shoulders, you will unconsciously begin to hold your shoulders in a dropped, relaxed position when standing in your normal posture.

DESCRIPTION

From an erect stance, hands down by your sides, bring up both shoulders as if you wanted to cover your ears. Then begin rotating your shoulders backwards, down, and forwards in a complete circle. Reverse the direction of the roll for another complete circle.

NUMBER OF REPETITIONS

Beginner: 8 rotations forward; 8 rotations backwards
Intermediate: 12 rotations in each direction
Advanced: 16 rotations in each direction

COUNT

This exercise should be done to a count of 4.

1. up
2. back
3. down
4. return to center

EFFECTS

This exercise will help you gain the full range of motion in the shoulder, and strengthen the muscles for punches, blocks, etc. It will also greatly improve your posture by properly aligning your shoulders to the rest of your body. Your chest will be up and out, and your shoulders will be dropped and relaxed.

SHOULDER ROLL

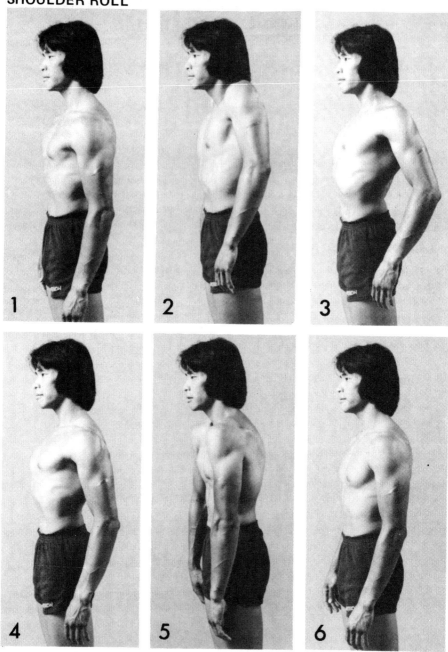

1. Begin in an erect stance, hands down by your sides.
2. Bring up both shoulders as if you wanted to cover your ears.
3. Begin rotating your shoulders back...
4. Then down...
5. Forward...
6. And finally return to the original position.

BACKWARDS ARM SWING

Shoulder muscles tend to hold more tension than other muscles and must be limbered continuously. Try this exercise when you feel stiff from sitting in one place for too long a time.

DESCRIPTION

Stand erect with your right foot forward at a 45 degree angle. Ease your weight on to the right toe. Your right heel will be slightly off the floor. Swing both arms back over your head with a firm swing. Do not jerk your shoulders. Lock your pelvis and arch your lower back as you swing. Then swing arms back to the starting position. You should first swing your arms straight back, then to the left (at a 45 degree angle) and finally to the right (at a 45 degree angle), alternating your feet respectively (i.e., left side, left foot turned at an angle).

NUMBER OF REPETITIONS

Beginner: 8 repetitions
Intermediate: 16 repetitions
Advanced: 24 repetitions

COUNT

This exercise should be done to a count of 6.

1. back swing, straight back
2. return to center
3. back swing to the left
4. return to center
5. back swing to the right
6. return to center

EFFECTS

This exercises all shoulder, upper back, and neck muscles. If done vigorously, it will stretch the lower back muscles. By arching the back, you will stretch and strengthen the upper abdominal muscles as well.

BACKWARDS ARM SWING

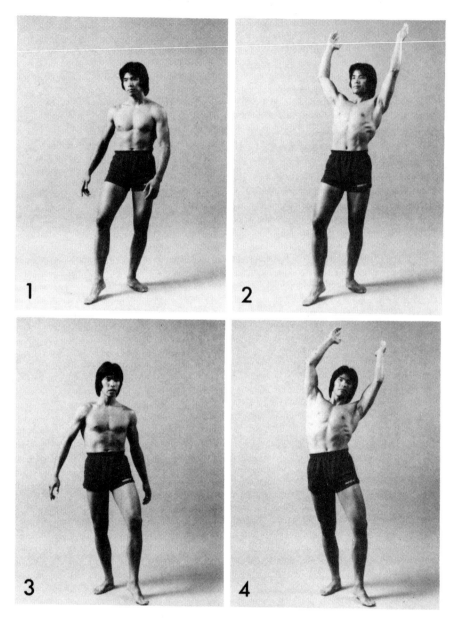

1. Stand erect with your right foot forward at a 45 degree angle, and your weight on your right toe.
2. Begin swinging both arms back. While swinging your arms, lock your pelvis and arch your lower back.
3. After returning to your original position, put your left foot forward and put your weight on your left toe.
4. Again swing both arms back.

CONCENTRATED PUSH-UPS

The traditional push-up is a powerful conditioner for all of your upper torso and shoulder muscles. It involves generally all of the upper body muscles to some extent.

DESCRIPTION

Lie face down, legs extended. You may put your feet on a chair. Place your palms directly under your shoulders. Do not raise your head, but concentrate on keeping your backbone straight. Push up, lifting your entire body off the floor. Do not let your upper body form an angle with your legs, but keep your body as straight as possible. When you reach the full extension of the arms (elbows should be locked out), slowly sink back down. Do not fall back, but feel your muscles resisting the pull of gravity. Barely touch the ground before pushing up again. This push-up differs from the regular push-up in that it is done very slowly. You should feel every muscle at work, with your mind remaining alert and calm.

NUMBER OF REPETITIONS

Beginner: 8 repetitions
Intermediate: 16 repetitions
Advanced: 24 repetitions

COUNT

This exercise should be done to a count of 6.

1, 2, 3. upward motion
4, 5, 6. downward motion

VARIATIONS

1. Experiment with placing your palms at different heights along your body. For example, place your palms at shoulder level; place your palms at chest level.

2. Experiment with placing your palms at different widths. For example, place your palms at shoulder width; then place your palms together so they are touching beneath your body.

3. Experiment with fist push-ups, which develop the wrist and improve positioning for punching correctly.

4. Experiment with one handed push-ups to intensify the conditioning of each arm.

EFFECTS

By trying all the variations of this exercise, you can concentrate its effects on different muscle groups. This specificity will help you become aware of the relationship of strength, coordination, and balance in your body.

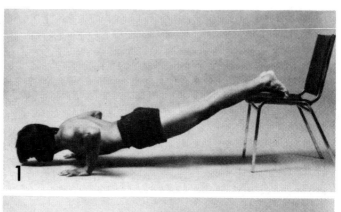

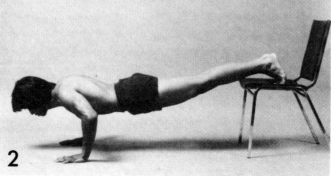

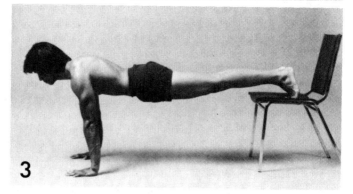

1. Lie face down, legs extended, with your feet on a chair.
2. Push up, lifting your entire body off the floor.
3. Reach the full extension of your arms, but do not lock your elbows.

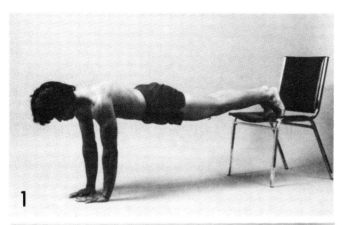

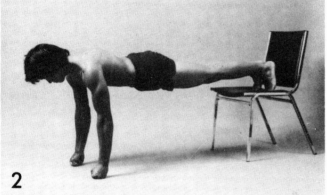

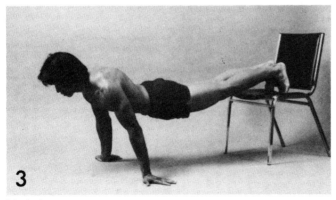

Variations
1. Place your hands so they are touching each other.
2. Experiment with fist push-ups.
3. Place your hands at shoulder width.

CONCENTRATED SIT-UPS

This variation of a classic exercise should be a part of every strengthening routine.

DESCRIPTION

Lie on the floor with legs bent. Cross one leg over the other. Drop your chin to your chest and put your hands at your waist. Carefully curl up at a slow rate until your lower back is barely touching the floor. Never jerk the torso upward. When you have reached the height of the sit-up, pause and curl back down very slowly. Much of the work done by the abdominals is done on the backwards roll when you are resisting gravity.

NUMBER OF REPETITIONS

Beginner: 10 repetitions
Intermediate: 20 repetitions
Advanced: 30 or more repetitions.

COUNT

This exercise should be done to a count of 6.

1, 2, 3. curling up
4, 5, 6. curling back

EFFECTS

Sit-ups are particularly valuable for strengthening the iliopsoas abdominal muscles, which hold the internal organs. As the muscles of the abdomen support the middle of your body and help draw up your legs, the exercise increases flexibility as well as strength.

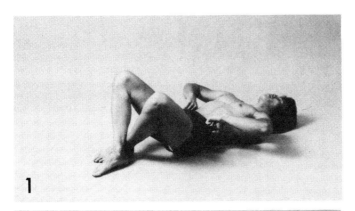

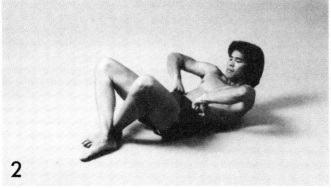

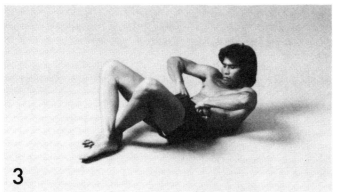

1. Lie on the floor with knees bent, one ankle crossed over the other.
2. Begin slowly curling up, keeping your elbows bent and your hands on your waist.
3. Continue to curl until the lower back is barely touching the floor.

KNEE BENDS

Deep knee bends, which require that you sink all the way down to rest on your heels, have recently been found to put unnecessary additional stress on the kneecaps. Partial knee bends, however, are excellent exercises for lubricating the knee joints and strengthening the muscles around the knee. Remember not to sink down past a sitting position when practicing this exercise. Thighs should remain parallel to the floor.

DESCRIPTION

Stand erect with legs at shoulder width. Put your hands palms down, straight out in front of you for balance. Bend your knees slowly until your thighs are parallel to the floor. Be rooted, and keep the soles of your feet on the floor during the entire exercise.

Do not jerk the knee, either when coming to a stop or when beginning to rise from the bend. The motion must be smooth and slow.

NUMBER OF REPETITIONS

Beginner: 8 repetitions
Intermediate: 16 repetitions
Advanced: 24 repetitions

COUNT

In this exercise, hold the bend for a count of 5.

EFFECTS

After practicing this exercise, you will find that your knee is able to come up unusually quickly for a kick or block.

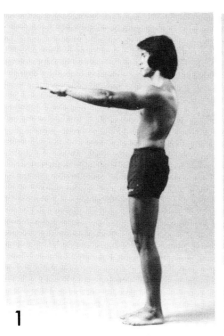

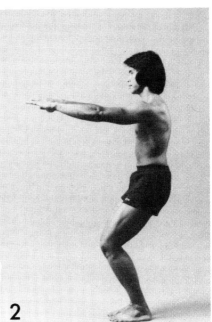

1

2

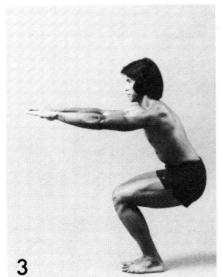

3

1. Stand erect, with legs at shoulder width. Extend your arms
straight out in front of you, palms down.
2. Begin to bend your knees slowly.
3. Continue bending your knees until your thighs are parallel to the
floor.

KNEE LIFTS

DESCRIPTION

Stand erect with feet shoulder width apart, knees slightly bent. Put arms in front of you, elbows bent, fingers lightly laced together. Your arms form a flat plane which will measure the distance your knees must rise. Quickly and evenly, maintaining a balanced posture, bring your knee up to the point where your hands are clasped. Return quickly by relaxing and dropping your foot. Repeat with the other leg.

NUMBER OF REPETITIONS

Beginner: 8 repetitions
Intermediate: 16 repetitions
Advanced: 24 repetitions

COUNT

This exercise should be done to a count of 2.

1. upward movement
2. downward movement

VARIATION

Beginner: Hold clasped hands below the waist
Intermediate: Hold clasped hands at the waist
Advanced: Hold clasped hands at mid or upper torso

EFFECTS

This exercise is especially valuable for strengthening the quadriceps muscles (front of thigh) and in improving your balance. Like the knee bends, it also improves the speed with which you are able to snap your knee up for blocks and kicks. Your recovery rate will also be enhanced.

1. Stand erect with feet shoulder width apart, knees slightly bent. Put your arms in front of you, elbows bent, fingers lightly laced together.
2. Shift your weight onto your right leg, and begin bringing your left knee up.
3. As you raise your knee, maintain a balanced posture.
4. Continue raising your knee until it reaches the plane made by your clasped hands.

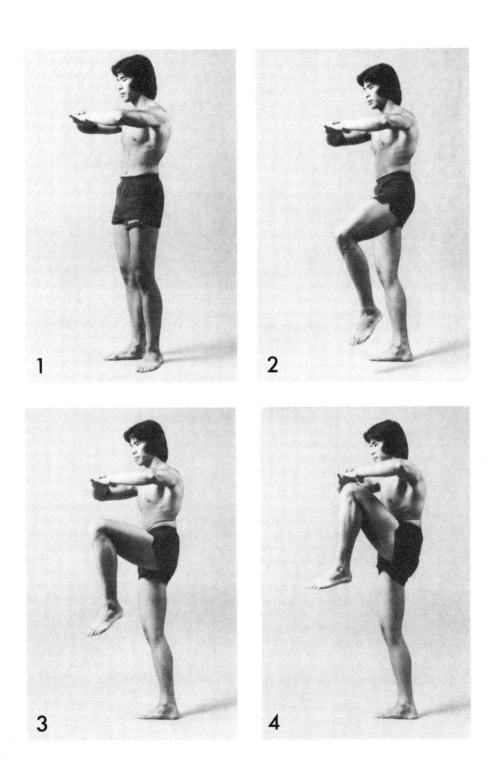

45

Dynamic Strength Exercises

The following exercises are designed to strengthen every muscle group in your body. Closely observe the photos while reading the text, noting the body positions and the muscles being flexed. The first time you do each exercise, slowly follow the directions and carefully compare your movements to those in the photo. It is vital to do each exercise correctly in order to get its full benefit.

You will see that each dynamic strength exercise is actually a simple series of motions which pits muscle against muscle. Each muscle is resisting, yet yielding at the same time. Since every muscle in your body is matched by another muscle or group of muscles, your body will be strengthened evenly and naturally.

In dynamic strength, muscles can be isolated and separately strenghtened. This selectivity factor makes it an excellent part of a training program. Deficiencies in specific areas can be eliminated by concentrating on the exercises for those respective muscles.

Most people are unaware of the total potential of which their bodies are capable. In a sense, the dynamic strength program is a process of continuing self-discovery which encourages individual experimentation in order to discover new facts about one's physical being. The goal of each session should be to gain some new understanding, some previously unknown information about how your body functions and its range of possibilities. Only through such exploration can you stimulate your body's untapped resources to extend beyond your current limitations and reach new heights of physical accomplishment. Through the discipline of dynamic tension exercises, you will be able to strengthen your muscles, increase power and improve your physique.

COMPLETE UPPER TORSO CONDITIONING

The upper torso consists of the shoulder muscles (deltoids), the chest muscles (pectorals), upper back (trapezius), lower back (latissimus dorsi), abdomen, and arm muscles. The following exercises use dynamic tension to condition and strengthen many of these important muscle groups at the same time, providing an even conditioning for your entire upper body.

DRY LAND SWIMMING

DESCRIPTION

Stand erect with feet shoulder width apart, knees slightly bent. The left hand should be palm up at your side; the right arm should be extended straight forward at chest level. Bring the right arm to the side, slowly shifting it from a palm down to a palm up position. As you bring the arm down, begin to slowly move the left arm back, up, and over in a swimming movement. Slowly turn the arm from a palm up to a palm down position. The left arm should be completely palm down at the end of the movement. The right arm should be in a palm up position when it reaches your side. Continue this slow circular movement. It is much like swimming, except the amount of tension generated in your arms is much greater.

NUMBER OF REPETITIONS

> **Beginner:** 3 repetitions
> **Intermediate:** 6 repetitions
> **Advanced:** 9 repetitions

COUNT

The movement of one arm from palm up position to palm down position should take four slow counts.

EFFECTS

As in regular swimming, this exercise affects the chest, shoulders, upper back, and arms. The deltoids (shoulder muscles) will undergo particularly intensive strengthening.

MARTIAL ARTS BENEFITS

Increased strength in this area can be demonstrated in a finger jab, which you will be able to deliver with much greater power. The forward motion of this exercise can be used in sinking hand movements. If you block a chest blow downwards with a hard fast movement, you will send all of your energy downwards as well. If you have control in your elbows and deltoids, you will be able to let your arm sink down forward just far enough to deflect the blow and then move up for an attack with a finger jab.

1. Stand erect, with the left hand palm up at your side and the right arm extended straight forward at chest level.
2. Begin moving the right arm to your side, slowly shifting to a palm up position. At the same time, slowly move the left arm back and up.
3. Continue moving your left arm up and over in a swimming motion.
4. At the end of the movement, your left arm is palm down in front of you; the right arm is palm up at your side. Continue this swimming movement.

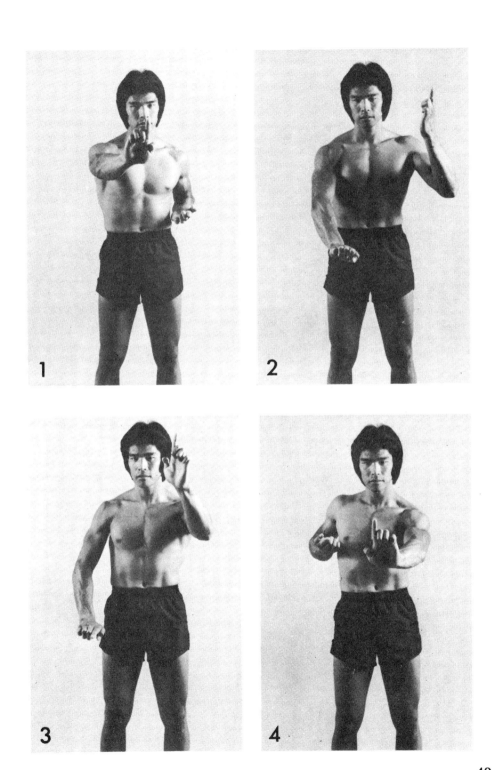

DRY LAND SWIMMING

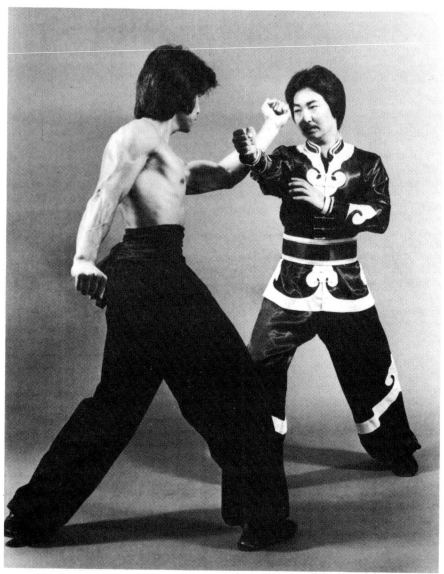

Use the increased strength in the deltoids, biceps, and forearms to develop control in your blocks and strikes. Let your arm sink forward only far enough to deflect the blow; then transform the downward energy into an upward attack to the temple.

VERTICAL PALM PRESS

DESCRIPTION

Stand erect with feet shoulder width apart, knees slightly bent. Bring your arms up to waist level, elbows bent. Now with palms facing forward, push out as slowly as possible and with as much tension as possible. Imagine you are pushing a huge, heavy object. You may find your muscles slightly shaking from the extreme tension you are generating. When you reach full extension—elbows locked—slowly return to the original position.

NUMBER OF REPETITIONS

Beginner: 3 repetitions
Intermediate: 6 repetitions
Advanced: 9 repetitions

COUNT

This exercise should be done to a count of 6 or more.

1, 2, 3. arms reaching full extension
1, 2, 3. arms returning to their original position

VARIATIONS

Perform the push at eye level and chest level as well as at waist level. Put both arms behind the small of your back, palms facing backwards (away from your body) and press backwards.

EFFECTS

This exercise provides intensive conditioning for the upper and lower back muscles and for all of the muscles in the upper arm, forearm, hands, and wrists.

MARTIAL ARTS BENEFITS

This will give you the power to make short punches without using the waist as the axis. You will be able to use the muscles from the back, shoulders, and arms to deliver a short but extremely powerful snap. The variations of this exercise will develop your ability to deliver this snap from various angles. Practicing at the waist level gives the power for take down palm thrusts to the pelvic area. Practice in pushing behind the back will help you to inflict sharp pain to the groin area when an opponent tries for an arm lock from behind.

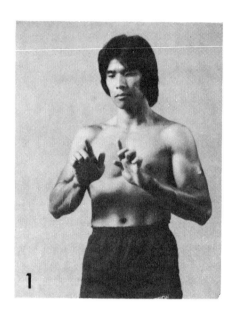

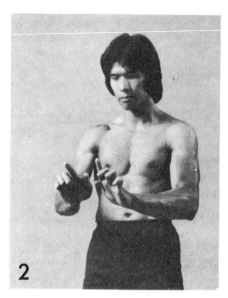

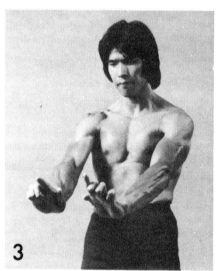

1. Stand erect, arms at waist level, with palms facing forward.
2. Begin pushing out as slowly as possible.
3. Continue pushing out until you reach full extension with elbows locked.

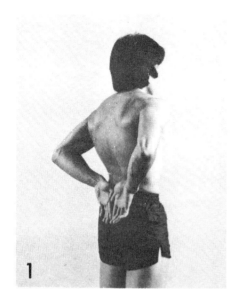

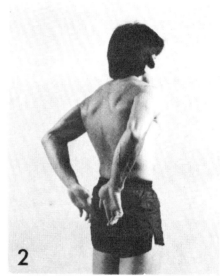

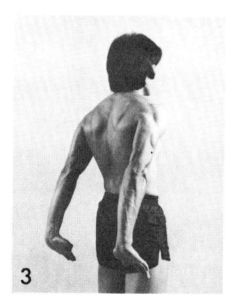

Variation
1. Stand erect, with both arms behind the small of your back,
palms facing backwards.
2. Slowly push backwards and down.
3. Continue pushing until you reach full extension.

VERTICAL PALM PRESS

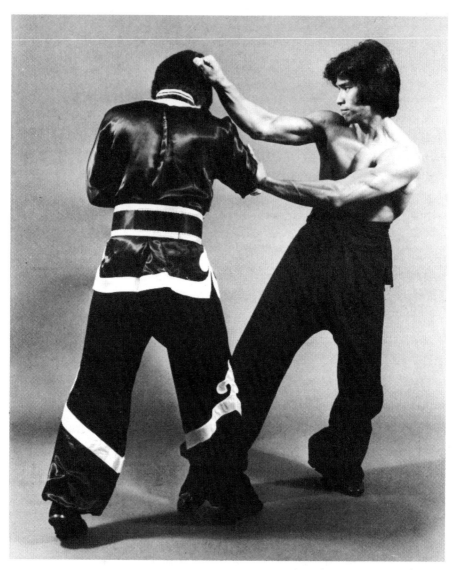

By developing strong back, shoulder, and arm muscles, you will be able to deliver a short, powerful snap to the back of your opponent's head without using your waist as an axis.

CHAIR DIPS

DESCRIPTION

Position yourself between two chairs placed about two feet apart. Lower yourself to the floor, supporting your weight by placing your hands on the chairs. Your legs are outstretched, supported by your heels. Continue lowering yourself until you barely touch the floor. Then push yourself up to the full extension of your arms. Keep head up and back straight while relaxing your shoulders.

NUMBER OF REPETITIONS

Beginner: 5 repetitions
Intermediate: 10 repetitions
Advanced: 15 repetitions

COUNT

This exercise should be done to a count of 6.

1, 2, 3. lowering movement
4, 5, 6. raising movement

VARIATIONS

Experiment with the position of your hands on the chairs. Try pointing your fingers forward, then at a 45 degree angle to the right; finally at a 45 degree angle to the left.

EFFECTS

This is a complete strengthener of the upper body, exercising the arms, shoulders, chest, and all of the back muscles.

MARTIAL ARTS BENEFITS

By concentrating on strengthening your arms, you will develop the versatility to strike in all directions. You may find that you can surprise your opponent by executing powerful palm strikes behind your back. Floor attacks can be enhanced by supporting your body with your hands, pushing off at the moment of execution.

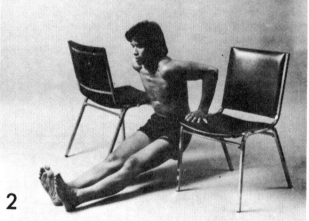

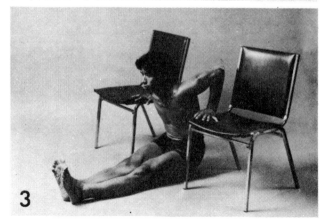

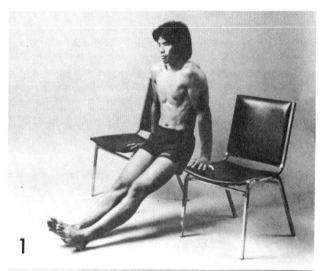

CHAIR DIPS

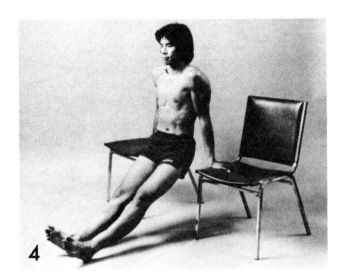

1. Position yourself between two chairs placed about two feet apart.
2. Lower yourself to the floor, supporting your weight by placing your hands on the chairs.
3. Continue to lower yourself until you barely touch the floor.
4. Then push yourself back up to the full extension of your arms.

DON'T bend your upper torso forward as you push up. Keep your back straight throughout the exercise.

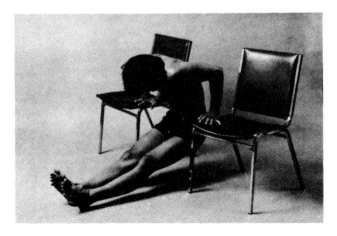

CHAIR DIPS

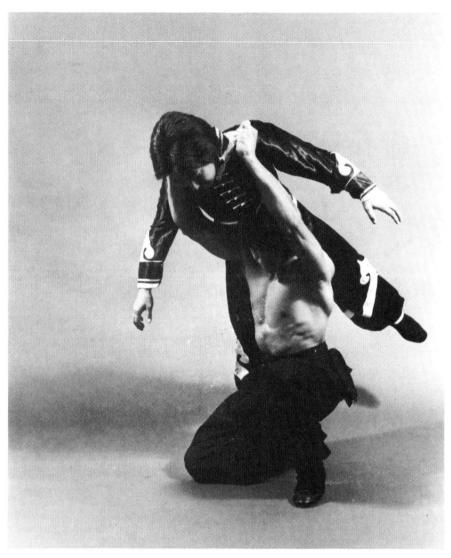

The development of powerful upper arm and shoulder muscles is vital for effective throws and takedowns.

UPPER TORSO—CHEST CONDITIONERS

The chest muscles are divided into two groups, the pectoralis minor (the smaller upper pectoral) and the pectoralis major (the large lower pectoral). The following exercises provide especially intensive conditioning for these areas.

PRAYER PRESS

DESCRIPTION

Stand erect with feet shoulder width apart, knees slightly bent. Extend arms straight out, palms together. Press the palms together exerting as much force as possible. Slowly bring the palms inward until your wrists touch your breast bone. Continue to exert maximum pressure through the entire movement while resisting the inward pull. When the praying hands have reached your chest, rotate the fingers upwards until the thumbs are touching the breast bone. Then rotate the praying hands downward until the little fingers are pointing down. Return the praying hands to the center position, and begin returning to the outstretched posture pushing out.

NUMBER OF REPETITIONS

Beginner: 3 repetitions
Intermediate: 6 repetitions
Advanced: 9 repetitions

COUNT

This exercise should be done to a count of 5.

1, 2. inward movement
3. hands rotate up
4. hands rotate down
5. return to starting position

EFFECTS

This exercise is a powerful strengthener of the pectoral muscles. It also strengthens the wrists, hands and fingers and tones the upper and lower back muscles.

MARTIAL ARTS BENEFITS

The upper body strength developed through this exercise will be invaluable in resisting and blocking body blows. In addition to its strengthening effect, the martial artist will find the praying position helpful in deflecting downward stick and hammer-like blows.

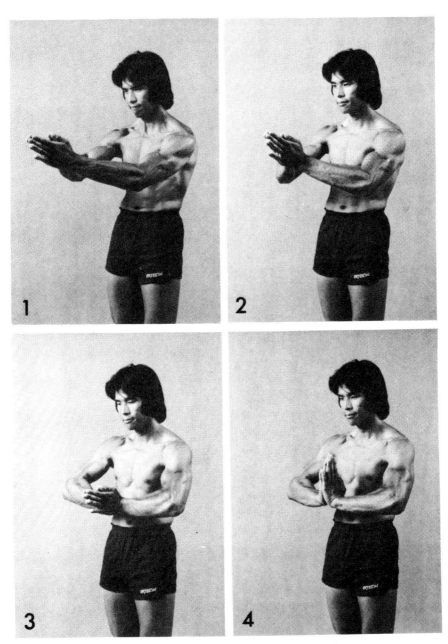

1. Stand erect, with arms extended straight out, palms together.
2. Press the palms together as you begin moving the palms inward.
3. Exert maximum pressure as you bring the palms in to touch your breast bone.
4. When the praying hands have reached your chest, rotate the fingers upwards until the thumbs are touching the breast bone.

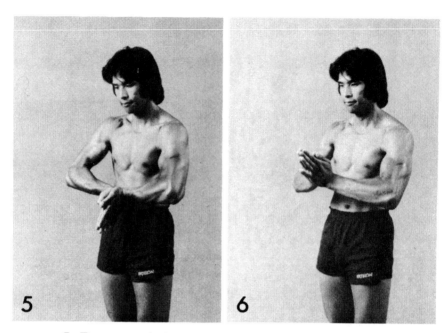

5. Then rotate the hands downward until the little fingers are pointing down.

6. Return the praying hands to the center position and begin moving forwards to the original position.

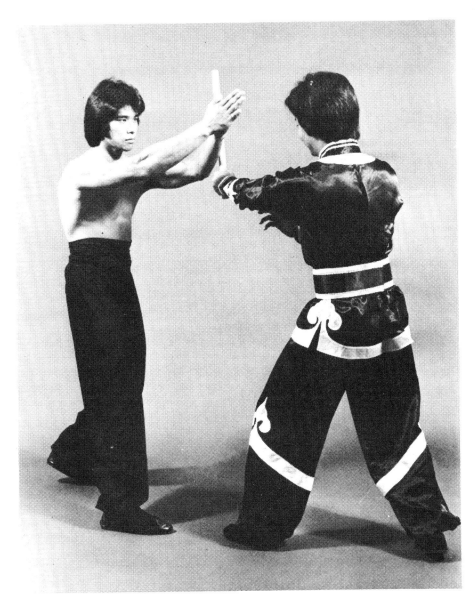

Brace your arms in the prayer press position to deflect stick attacks.

CROSSING HANDS

DESCRIPTION

Stand erect with feet shoulder width apart, knees slightly bent, arms at your side. Bring your arms up to chest level, elbows bent and pressed back. Slowly move your arms towards each other, resisting the movement of the triceps with the contraction of the biceps. As your arms come closer, cross your right arm over your left, and arch your back to feel the tension in your pectorals and abdominals. (You should feel tension through your pectoral muscles, arms, hands, and fingers.)

NUMBER OF REPETITIONS

Beginner: 3 repetitions
Intermediate: 6 repetitions
Advanced: 9 repetitions

COUNT

This exercise should be done to a count of 2.

1. upward motion
2. downward motion

VARIATIONS

1. Cross your arms at eye level; shoulder level; and waist level. This strengthens the different levels of the pectoral muscles.
2. Standing in a horse stance with your knees bent, shift your weight onto the right leg. Seventy percent of your weight should be on the right leg, thirty percent on the left leg. Cross your hands from this position. Then shift the weight in your legs, and cross your hands from the new position. This will strengthen your arms and torso for varying the angles of attack. Strength comes from the additional flexibility gained by the stretching elements of this exercise.

EFFECTS

This exercise strengthens the abdominals, chest, triceps, and biceps. The triceps receive an especially concentrated workout.

MARTIAL ARTS BENEFITS

Triceps are called into play for any movement which requires pushing with the arms. This means that any outward block or punch would benefit from increased power in the triceps.

You will find that with strong triceps, you will be able to get more of a thrust in your punches. For example, you may use the forearm and elbow to push out for a punch. At the last minute, add an extra thrust with the triceps, so that the force is intensified by a whipping snap. Always remember to explode through your target when punching.

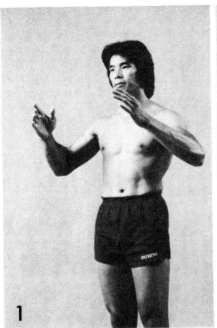

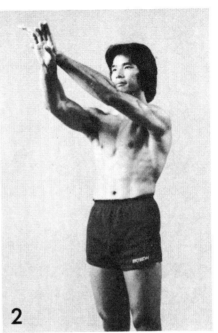

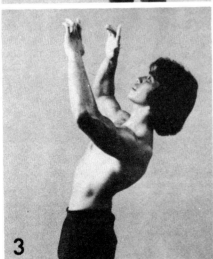

1. Bring your arms up to chest level, elbows bent and back.
2. Slowly move your arms toward each other.
3. As you cross your right arm over your left, arch your back to feel tension in your pectorals and abdominals.

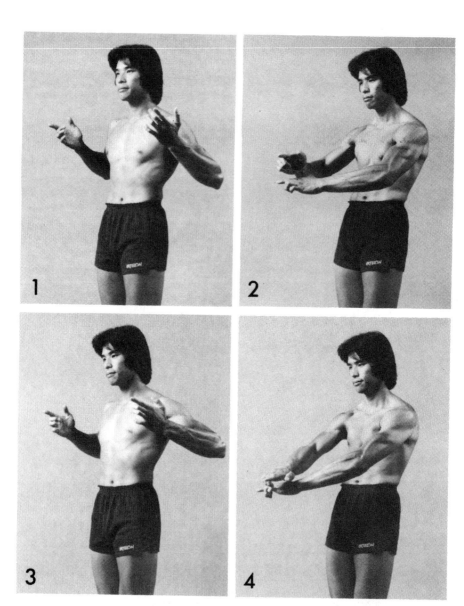

Variation
1. Bring your arms up to chest level.
2. As you move your arms towards each other, angle them slightly downwards so they cross at waist level.
3. Bring your arms back up to chest level.
4. This time, cross your arms below waist level.

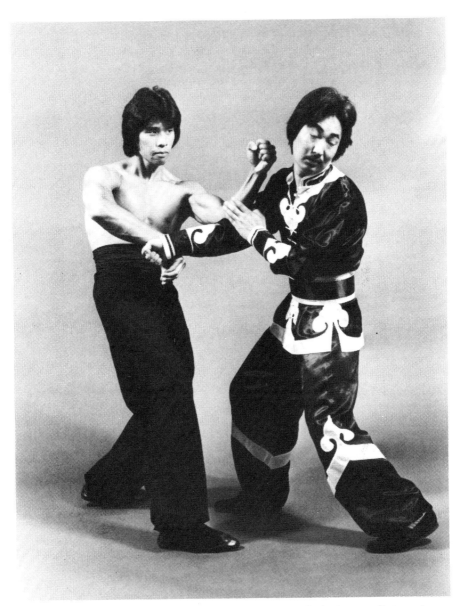

Strong triceps are essential for snapping a punch through the target. Outward blocks also benefit from increased power in the triceps.

T.N.T.

DESCRIPTION

Stand erect with feet shoulder width apart, knees slightly bent. Begin bringing both arms up to shoulder level, keeping your elbows slightly lower than your shoulders. With fists closed, push down slowly, resisting the downward push of the triceps. Continue the movement to waist level. At the moment of completion, bend your knees. You should feel tension in your pectorals, deltoids, hands and arms.

NUMBER OF REPETITIONS

Beginner: 3 repetitions
Intermediate: 6 repetitions
Advanced: 9 repetitions

COUNT

This exercise should be done to a count of 4.

1, 2. upward motion
3, 4. downward motion

VARIATIONS

1. Turn your body from side to side, pushing down at a 45 degree angle.
2. Cross your hands while performing the exercise.
3. Open and close your hands.

EFFECTS

This exercise strengthens and stretches the abdominals, chest, arm and triceps muscles. In the first variation, the waist also is emphasized.

MARTIAL ARTS BENEFITS

Performing the T.N.T. exercise will greatly benefit coordination of double hand blows. The sinking action which occurs by bending the knees uses your body weight to unbalance your opponent. This sinking technique is the correct method of executing all take downs and throws.

1. Stand erect with feet shoulder width apart, knees slightly bent.
2. Begin raising both arms. As your arms reach shoulder level, elbows slightly lower than your shoulders, clench your hands in fists.
3. Begin to push down with your fists, resisting the downward push of the triceps.
4. Continue the pushing motion until you reach waist level. At the moment of completion, bend your knees.

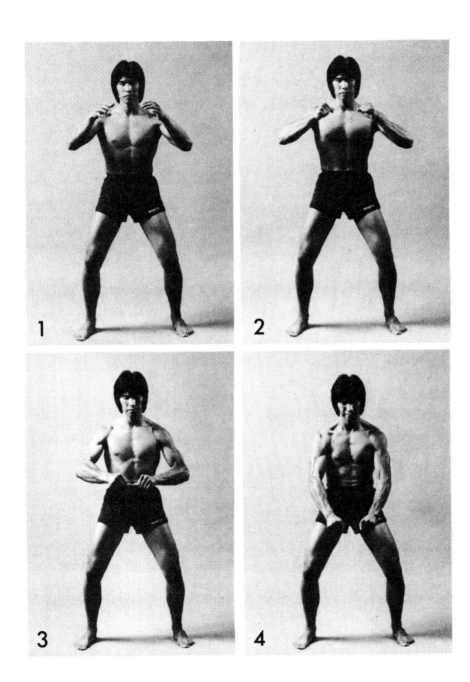

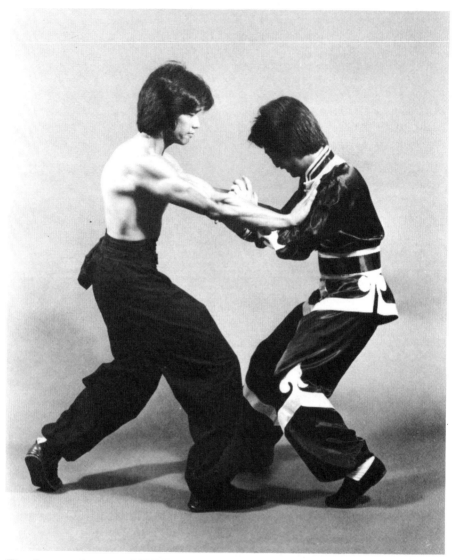

The downward power of T.N.T., strengthening the pectorals, deltoids, hands and arms, is effective in double hand blows. Note how the knees bend and the torso sinks to focus the power of the entire body behind the blow.

WHISKING ARMS

DESCRIPTION

Stand erect with feet together, hands at your sides. Cross your arms up in front of you, palms down, with your right arm under your left arm. (You should alternate this, with left arm under right arm.) Slowly but firmly throw your arms as far back as possible, feeling the stretch in the chest muscles, abdomen, and shoulders. As you do this exercise, note that the elbows move back first, then the forearm, and then the hands reach backwards in the final moment of the stretch. This backwards stretch should be performed at eye level, shoulder level, and waist level.

NUMBER OF REPETITIONS

Beginner: 8 repetitions
Intermediate: 16 repetitions
Advanced: 24 repetitions

COUNT

This exercise should be done to a slow count of 2.

1. throw arms back
2. return to starting position

VARIATIONS

In addition to varying the level at which the exercise is done, try positioning the hands with palms up to create tension in the bottom part of the arms, or in a fist to create tension in the forearm muscles.

EFFECTS

This exercise strengthens the wrists, forearms, biceps, triceps, pectorals, shoulder, upper back, and abdominal muscles.

MARTIAL ARTS BENEFITS

The whisking arms movements are called into play at three levels: at eye level, with knife edge chops to the temple; at shoulder level, with chops to the neck; and at waist level, with chops to the mid-section and groin. With strengthened chest muscles, your body will be able to deliver maximum power to a target at any of these three levels. Friction is greatly reduced by these exercises.

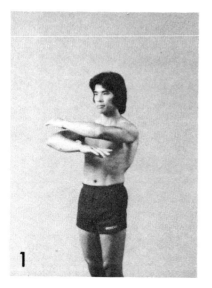

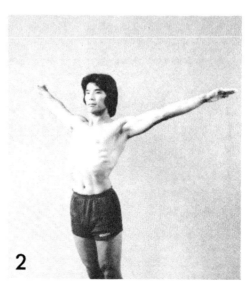

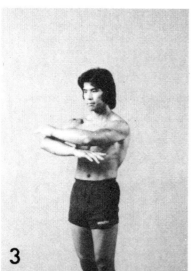

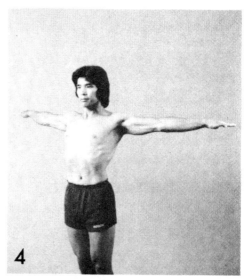

1. Stand erect, with feet together, arms crossed in front of you, palms down. Your right arm is under your left arm.
2. Throw your arms back as far as possible. Your outstretched hands should be at eye level.
3. Return your arms to the crossed position.
4. Swing your arms out at shoulder level.
5. Return your arms to the crossed position.
6. Swing your arms out at waist level.

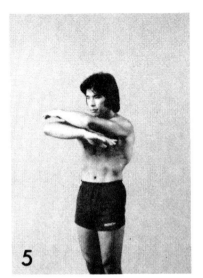
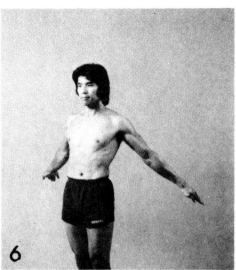
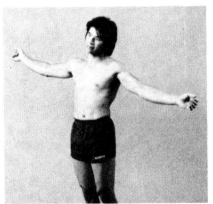

DON'T tilt your head to the side while swinging your arms back. Be sure to extend your arms fully in the final moment of stretch.

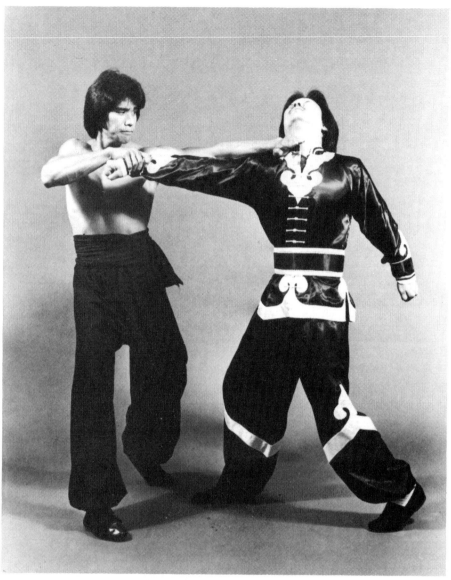

Power from the chest, back, and shoulders are focused through the left arm to deliver a stunning blow to the neck.

UPPER TORSO—WAIST CONDITIONERS

Waist exercises affect the muscles of the abdomen, lower back, hips, pelvic area, and buttocks. The twisting and bending exercises which follow are designed to increase both the strength and flexibility of these areas. You will find that maximum power is obtained when the limbs and waist are coordinated in all movements.

SIDE BENDS

DESCRIPTION

Sit in a chair, with feet shoulder width apart on the floor. Both arms should hang straight down at your sides. Imagine you are holding a heavy dumbbell on the right side. Slowly bring it down to the floor, stretching your waist muscles on the left side and contracting the waist muscles on the right side. Now, just as slowly, bring the imaginary dumbbell up. Do these side bends with a great deal of tension, as if lifting a heavy weight. Feel the stretch on the opposite side of the waist, the contraction in the lifting side of the waist, and the tension in your arm and shoulder muscles. Now do the same exercise with the left arm.

NUMBER OF REPETITIONS

Beginner: 5 repetitions with each arm
Intermediate: 10 repetitions with each arm
Advanced: 15 repetitions with each arm

COUNT

This exercise should be done to a count of 3.

1, 2. downward movement
3. upwards movement

The downward pull is very important in providing a stretch and contraction of the waist muscles.

EFFECTS

This exercise is particularly good for strengthening the arm and waist muscles. It also encourages flexibility in the waist.

MARTIAL ARTS BENEFITS

The combination of flexibility and strength from this exercise will give you precise control over your movements when you evade and counter a punch.

1. Sit in a chair with feet shoulder width apart, arms straight down at your sides.
2. Slowly bring your right arm down to the side, as if it were holding a heavy weight.
3. Return to your original position, and then slowly bring your left arm all the way down.

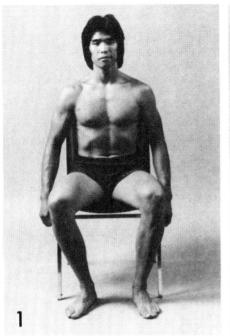

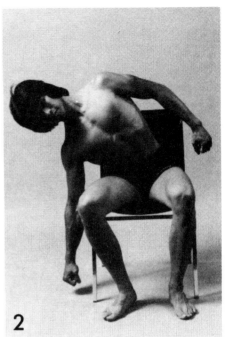

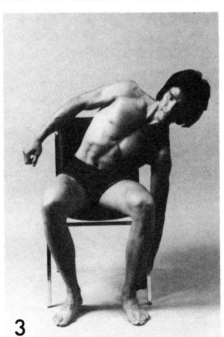

SIDE BENDS

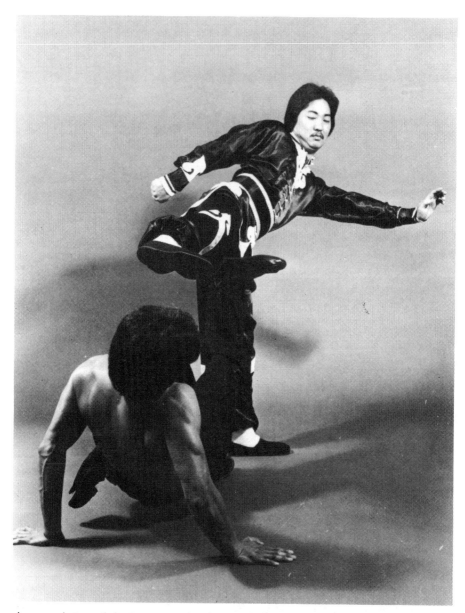

Increased strength in the arm and waist muscles promotes the flexibility and speed necessary for dodging blows and kicks.

TORSO TWISTING

DESCRIPTION

Stand in the horse stance, with feet approximately four feet apart. Raise your arms to the side at shoulder level. Lock your pelvis in position, then twist your body slowly all the way to the left as far as it will go, resisting the movement as you turn. Then twist your upper body all the way to the right. Also maintain your head position, with the head looking straight ahead during the exercise. Using your arms for balance, put as much tension as possible into the sidewards movements.

NUMBER OF REPETITIONS

Beginner: 3 repetitions
Intermediate: 6 repetitions
Advanced: 9 repetitions

COUNT

This exercise should be done to a slow count of 2.

1. swing to the left
2. swing to the right

EFFECTS

This exercise will strengthen your waist, abdomen, pelvis, lower back, and pectorals.

MARTIAL ARTS BENEFITS

Power in every movement comes from the waist and hips. The waist is considered the big axis of power, while the limbs, palms, elbows, shoulders, knees, legs, ankles, etc. are considered the small axis. One turn of the big axis is equivalent to hundreds of turns of the small axis. Therefore, use of the waist's big movement produces more power than that produced by employing the limbs alone.

As this area increases in strength through movement, you will also find that when your opponent directs a blow to your body, you will be able to lean and turn with your body to avoid the punch and let it float by you. Your power will show itself not in resistance to the punch but in your control in evading it.

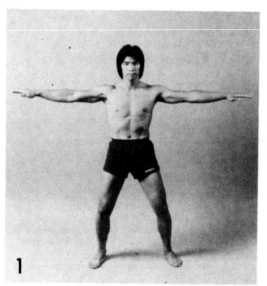
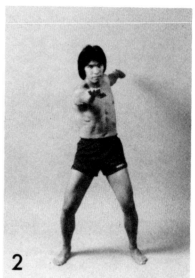
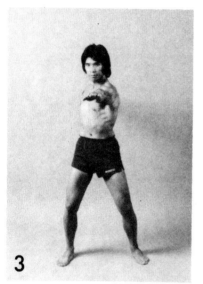
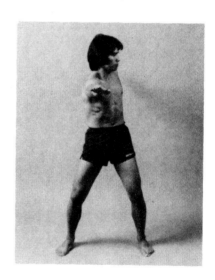

1. Stand in a horse stance, with arms extended to the side at shoulder level.

2. Lock your pelvis in position, then twist your body slowly all the way way to the left.

3. Then twist your body all the way to the right, as far as it will go.

DON'T turn your head to the side as your body is twisting. Your head should look straight ahead at all times.

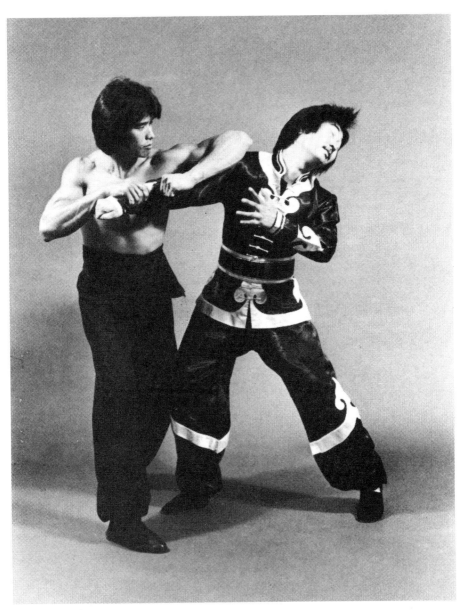

Twist the body to generate power from the pelvis and waist, focusing it in an effective blow to the head.

CONCENTRATED TWISTING

DESCRIPTION

Begin in a horse stance. Move your left arm up to the waist, elbow slightly bent, with the palm side of the hand up and your hand closed in a fist. As the left arm moves up to the waist, swing the right arm back behind your body with the palm down in a fist. As you bring your right fist back, and your left fist up, turn all the way to the right. Shift your weight slightly onto your right foot, but otherwise do not move your feet. When you have completed the right twist, begin turning to the left. As you turn to the left, bring the left fist back behind your body with your left fist palm down, and bring your right fist up to waist level with the fist palm up. Shift your weight lightly onto the left foot. Throughout this exercise, the pelvis should be locked so that all the twisting will be concentrated in the waist muscles. However, when you reach the extreme position of the twist, your pelvis should be already starting to move in the opposite direction for a smooth, gliding twist. There should be no jerks.

NUMBER OF REPETITIONS

Beginner: 5 repetitions in each direction
Intermediate: 10 repetitions in each direction
Advanced: 15 repetitions in each direction

COUNT

This exercise should be done to a count of 4.

1, 2. right twist
3, 4. left twist

EFFECTS

This strengthens the waist muscles, abdomen, lower back and shoulder muscles.

MARTIAL ARTS BENEFITS

By swinging slowly and using maximum concentration, you can greatly develop the power from the floor to your upper body. Using the pelvis as the axis of power, you will be able to put immense force behind your punches, and move with ease at the waist. Because this is a moving exercise, it also enhances your ability to evade punches with maximum control over your movement.

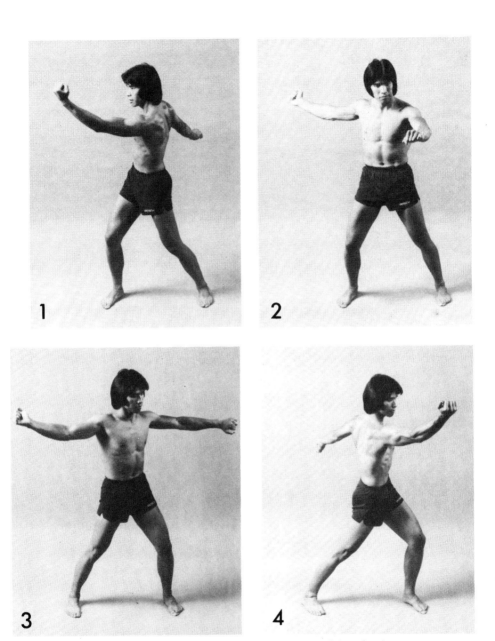

1. From the horse stance, turn all the way to the right. At the same time, swing the right fist back behind your body (palm down), and bring your left fist up to waist level (palm up).

2. When you have completed the right twist, begin turning left.

3. Continue the slow twist to the left.

4. When you reach the extreme position of the twist, your pelvis should already be moving in the opposite direction.

CONCENTRATED TWISTING

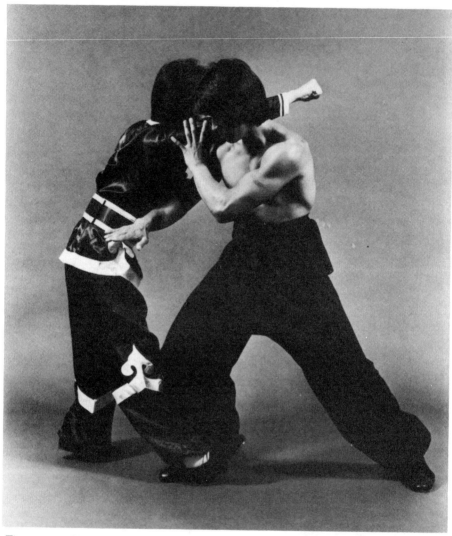

The power of the entire body, from the ground up through the legs, the torso, and into the arms, should be used to block a blow. The pelvis is used as the axis of power.

UPPER ARM CONDITIONERS

The upper arms, consisting of the biceps and triceps, are strengthened in most of the upper torso and chest conditioning exercises. The following exercises focus the dynamic tension for developing particularly powerful arms.

CURLS

DESCRIPTION

Stand erect, with feet shoulder width apart, knees slightly bent. Hold arms in front of you. With palms facing up, close your hands around an imaginary barbell or an ordinary stick. Begin slowly lifting your arms up, imagining that you are lifting an extremely heavy weight. Feel the tension in your arms, shoulders, and back as you lift it up. While lifting, be careful not to lean away, but keep your back straight. When you have lifted it as high as possible—fists should be close to your chest—begin slowly easing the imaginary weight downwards. Also be sure to reach the full extension of your arms in the downward motion.

NUMBER OF REPETITIONS

Beginner: 5 repetitions
Intermediate: 10 repetitions
Advanced: 15 repetitions

COUNT

This exercise should be done to a count of 4.

1,2. upwards movement
3,4. downwards movement

VARIATIONS

Try different grips on the imaginary barbell. For example, try a grip at shoulder width. Then try a close (hands together) grip.

EFFECTS

Both biceps and triceps are exercised here, the biceps on the upward movement and the triceps on the downward movement. By reaching your full extension in this exercise, you will increase the range of motion in the elbow joints and fully exercise the arm muscles.

MARTIAL ARTS BENEFITS

These exercises are excellent conditioners for any pulling, grabbing, choking, or general grappling technique that requires powerful arms. The variations on the exercise will tone all the different muscles in your shoulders, allowing you to use your pulling techniques from a variety of angles. Your muscles should feel looser, have more snap, and feel more springy than if the exercise were done with a weight.

1. Stand erect, feet shoulder width apart, knees slightly bent. With palms up, close your hand around a stick.
2. Begin slowly lifting your arms up, imagining you are lifting a heavy weight.
3. After you have lifted the stick as high as possible (fists close to chest), begin slowly easing the stick down.

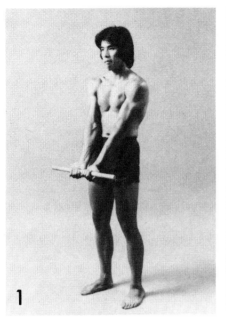

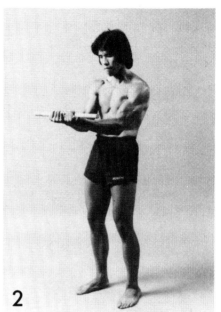

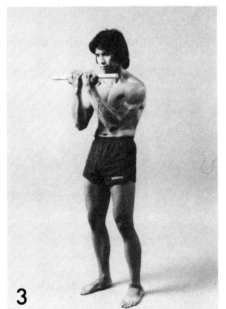

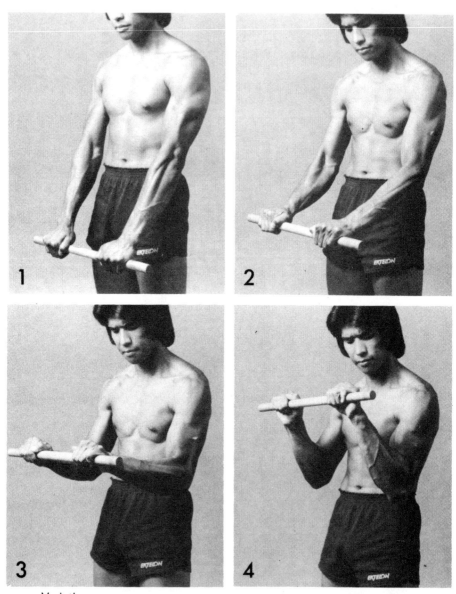

Variation
1. Hold the stick with your palms down, hands approximately six inches apart.
2. Begin slowly lifting your arms up.
3. As you lift, concentrate on feeling the maximum amount of tension in your arms.
4. Bring your arms as close to your chest as possible.

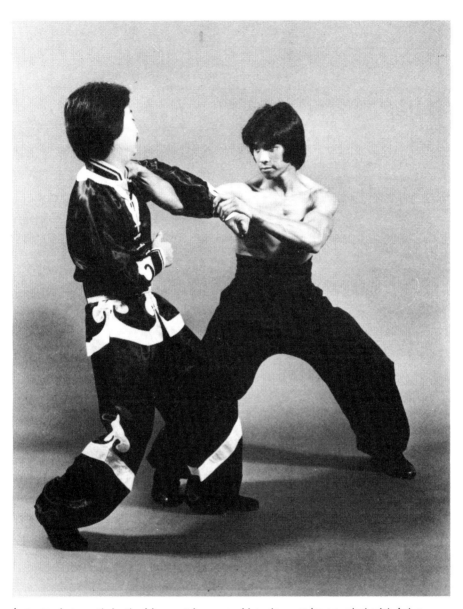

Increased strength in the biceps, triceps, and hands must be coupled with joint flexibility to intensify the effect of grabs.

FRENCH CURL

DESCRIPTION

Stand erect, with feet shoulder width apart, knees slightly bent. Start with arms down in front of you, palms down. Close your hands around an ordinary stick or an imaginary barbell. Then lift the barbell over your head, and bring it down to shoulder level behind your neck. Lift it up again until the barbell is above your head, then bring it down again to shoulder level. Continue this movement for the desired number of repetitions. (This is the same movement as for the standard french curl in weight training.)

NUMBER OF REPETITIONS

    Beginner: 5 repetitions
Intermediate: 10 repetitions
    Advanced: 15 repetitions

COUNT

This exercise should be done to a count of 4.

    1,2. bringing barbell down to neck
    3,4. lifting barbell above head

VARIATIONS

Hold the imaginary barbell at different widths, such as at shoulder width and with hands close together.

EFFECTS

The french curl is the basic triceps exercise. It also strengthens the biceps, shoulders, and upper back muscles.

MARTIAL ARTS BENEFITS

Triceps strength is needed in any martial arts technique calling for a quick upward movement of the arms and forearms, as in upward blocks or punches. Triceps are also used in pushing and throwing techniques.

1. Stand erect, feet shoulder width apart, knees slightly bent. Hold the stick over your head, arms extended but not locked.
2. Slowly bring the stick down to shoulder level behind your head.
3. Bring the stick as far behind your head as possible.

DON'T bend your head forward as you bring the stick down. Keep your head centered and upright at all times.

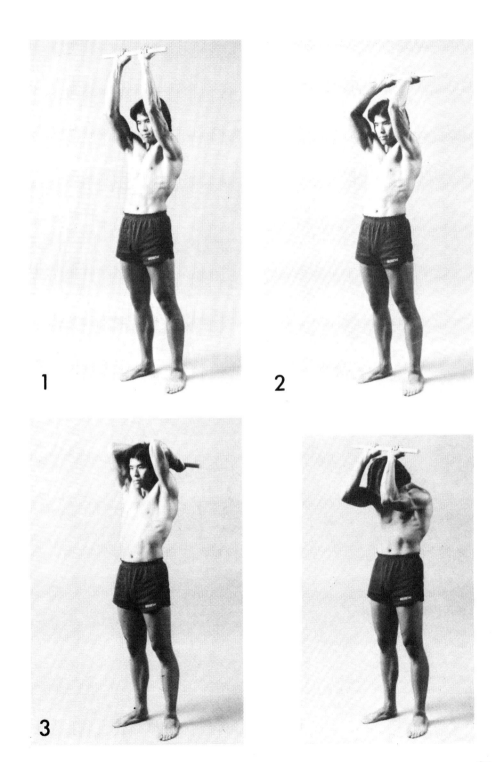

1

2

3

FRENCH CURL

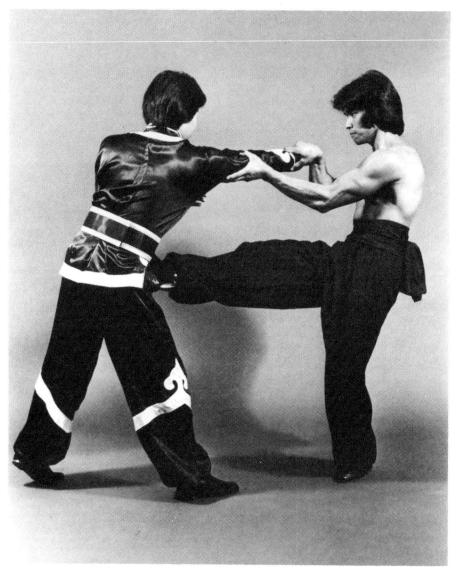

Triceps strength is vital in throwing techniques, allowing you to forcefully counter-balance your opponent's resistance.

PULLEYS

DESCRIPTION

Start in a horse stance. Put your left hand on your breast bone in the center of your chest. Extend your right arm at shoulder level. Begin pulling on an imaginary weight to bring your right arm to your chest. As you pull, feel the tension in your wrist, forearm, and biceps. When your right fist reaches your breast bone, reverse the motion. Now imagine that you are pulling a heavy weight from your chest, and slowly extend your arm. When you reverse the motion, you will feel increased tension in the triceps. Repeat this exercise with your left arm.

NUMBER OF REPETITIONS

Beginner: 5 repetitions
Intermediate: 10 repetitions
Advanced: 15 repetitions

COUNT

This exercise should be done very slowly, to a count of 5, to generate a great deal of tension.

EFFECTS

This exercise strengthens the wrists, biceps, triceps, shoulders, upper back, and chest muscles.

MARTIAL ARTS BENEFITS

The muscles strengthened by this exercise are particularly helpful in techniques requiring grabbing (pulling movements) as in a choke hold, or reverse movements as in a back fist.

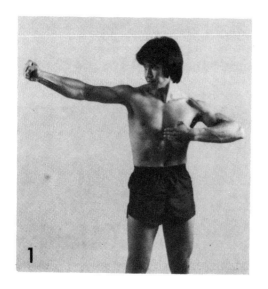 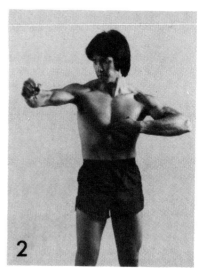

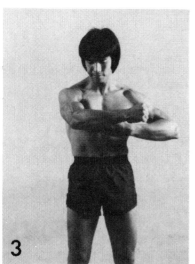 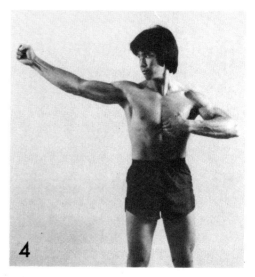

1. Starting in a horse stance, put your left hand on your breast bone and extend your right arm.
2. Begin pulling on an imaginary weight to bring your arm towards your your chest.
3. Continue the pulling motion until your right arm reaches your breast bone.
4. Then begin extending the arm, as if pulling the weight in the opposite direction.

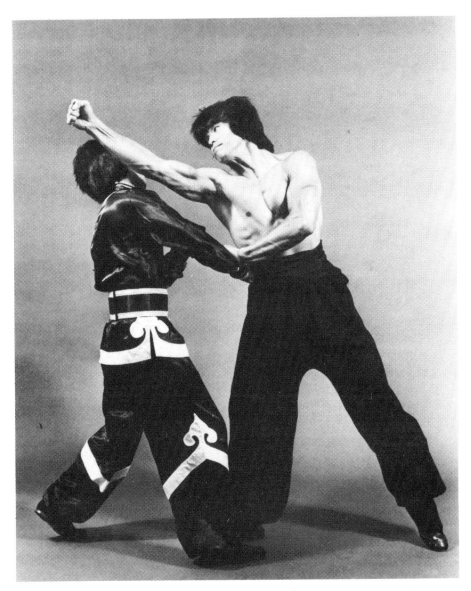

The pulleys develop the arm and back muscles necessary for devastating backfist blows.

FIST SALUTATION

DESCRIPTION

Stand in an erect stance, knees slightly bent. Put your arms in front of you across your body, with elbows bent, left fist inside of the right palm. Begin using the left fist to push the right arm across your body. At the same time, use your right arm to resist this push. When the right arm has reached its full extension across the body, the right open palm should begin to push the left fist across your body. Your elbows must always be lower than your fist.

NUMBER OF REPETITIONS

Beginner: 3 repetitions
Intermediate: 6 repetitions
Advanced: 9 repetitions

COUNT

This exercise should be done very slowly, using a count of 5.

EFFECTS

Like the pulleys, this exercise strengthens the chest muscles, arms, shoulders, and upper back muscles.

MARTIAL ARTS BENEFITS

The fist salutation is especially important in developing the punching power and correct positioning of the fist. It gives the martial artist the experience of driving through a target, and of exploding beyond even when the punch is smothered.

1. Stand erect with arms in front of you, elbows bent, left fist inside right palm.
2. Begin pushing the right arm across your body with the left fist.
3. Continue the pushing motion until the left arm has reached its full extension across the body.
4. Then begin using the right open palm to push the left fist across your body in the opposite direction.
5. Continue the pushing motion until the right arm has reached its full extension across the body.

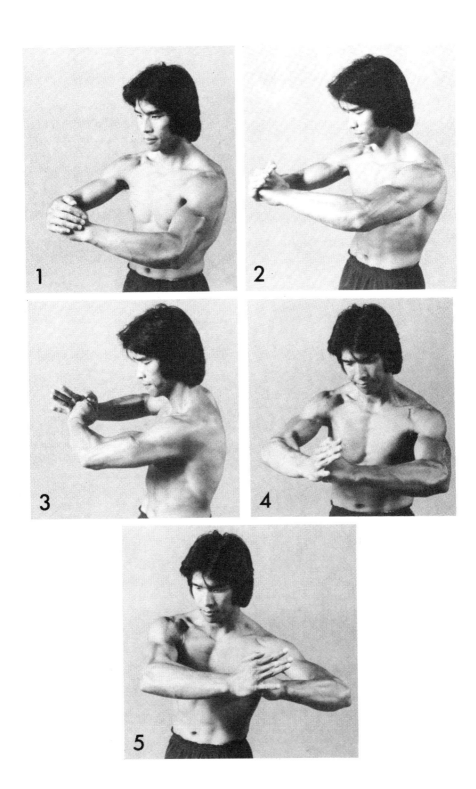

FIST SALUTATION

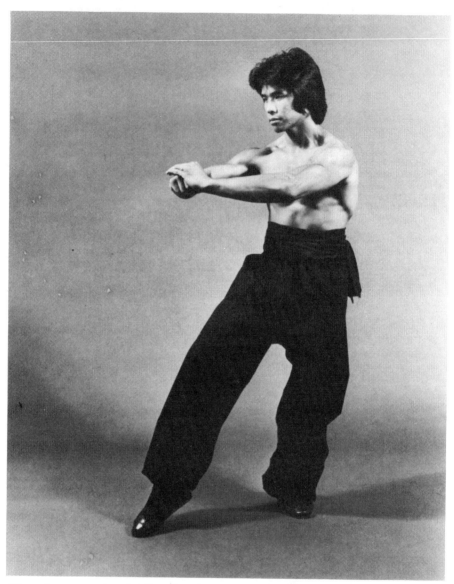

When done correctly, the fist salutation strengthens all of the muscles in the upper body, and locks into your muscles the sense of exploding beyond the target.

HAND AND FOREARM CONDITIONERS

No martial artist can ignore the importance of forearm and hand strength. However, most exercise programs neglect these important muscle groups. By emphasizing the following exercises in your workout, you should begin almost immediately to experience increased strength in your fingers, wrists, and all forearm muscles.

FINGER EXERCISES

DESCRIPTION

Stand erect, with feet shoulder width apart, knees slightly bent. Bring arms to waist level with elbows bent. Extend your hands with palms down. Slowly close your hand, starting with the index finger and curling all of your other fingers shut, one by one. Clench your hand in a fist, then begin opening the fist, starting from the little finger. When the hand is fully extended, begin the closing movement again. This exercise should be done by both hands, either one at a time, or both together.

NUMBER OF REPETITIONS

Beginner: 8 repetitions
Intermediate: 16 repetitions
Advanced: 24 repetitions

COUNT

This exercise should be done to a count of 6.

1,2,3. closing motion
4,5,6. opening motion

EFFECTS

All the small muscles in the fingers, wrists, and hands will be conditioned.

MARTIAL ARTS BENEFITS

The importance of strength in the fingers cannot be underestimated. Any hand move or technique using clawing, grabbing or pulling movements will benefit when you have the strength for vice-like locks and holds.

1. Extend your hands with palms down.
2. Slowly close your hand, starting with the index finger...
3. Then curl all of the fingers shut, one by one.
4. Clench your hand in a fist.
5. Then begin opening the fist, starting from the little finger...
6. Until the hand is fully extended.

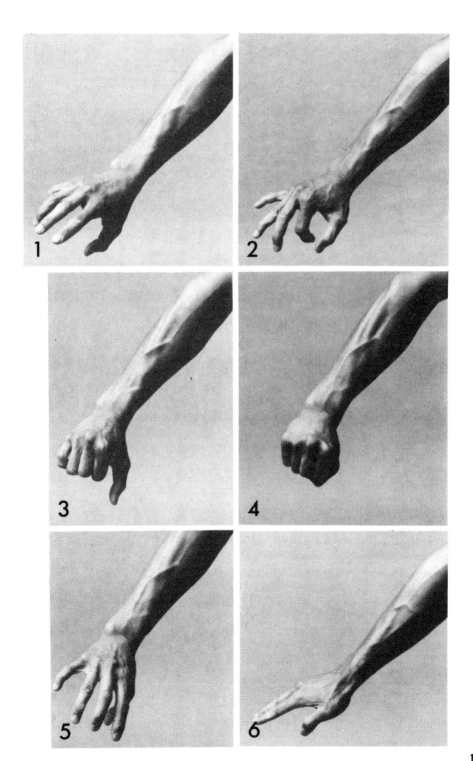

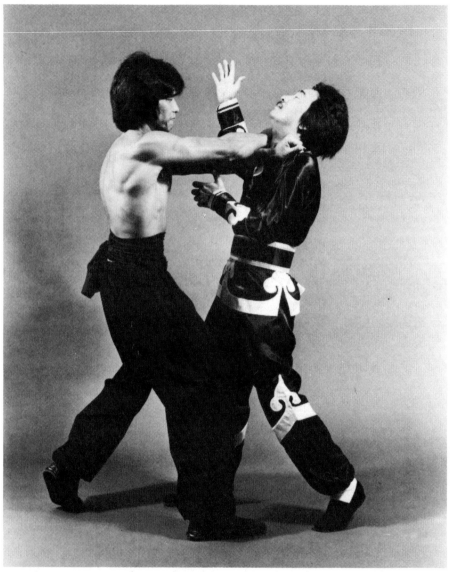

By increasing the strength in your fingers and hands you can make your blocking grabbing techniques maximally effective.

CRANE HAND

DESCRIPTION

Stand erect, with feet shoulder width apart, knees slightly bent. Bring one arm up to waist level. With your hand in a palm up position, fingers extended, pull your fingers toward you, pointing to your chest. Your wrist should be bent as far as possible so that your hand is at an acute angle to your forearm. Rotate your hand counter clockwise until your fingers point down and in toward your waist. In this end position, your fingers should be bent at an acute angle to the underside of your forearm. You should keep your arm stationary and feel the rotation only in your wrists. Now repeat the exercise using your other hand.

NUMBER OF REPETITIONS

    Beginner: 5 repetitions of each hand
Intermediate: 10 repetitions of each hand
    Advanced: 15 repetitions of each hand

COUNT

This exercise should be done to a count of 5.

EFFECTS

This exercise strengthens the fingers, hands, wrists, and forearms.

MARTIAL ARTS BENEFITS

Strength in the forearms and hands is especially helpful in hooking, striking, blocking, and evading wrist locks. Holds and jabs requiring finger strength are also benefited.

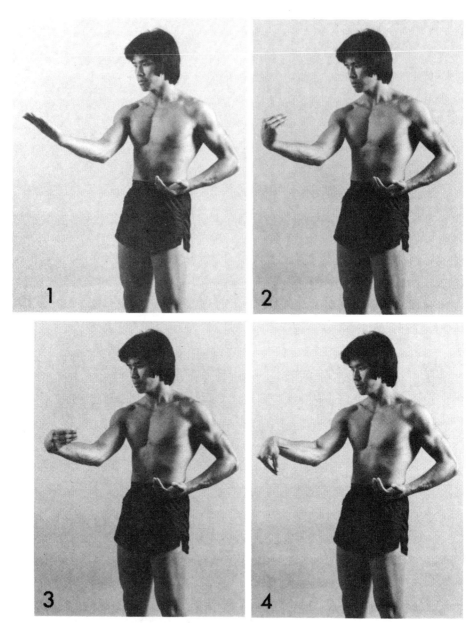

1. Stand erect, with your left arm at waist level, palm up.
2. Begin pulling your fingers up toward you, pointing to your chest.
3. When your wrist is bent as far as possible, begin rotating your hand counterclockwise.
4. Continue rotating until your fingers point down and in toward your waist.

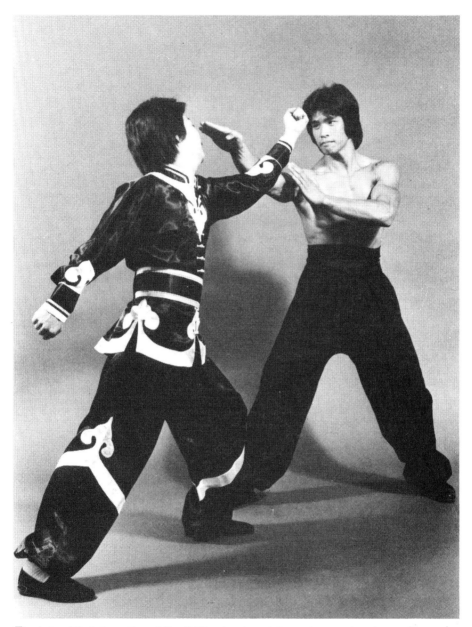

The intensified strength and flexibility developed through crane hand exercises makes the eye jab a devastating offensive technique.

WRIST ROLL

DESCRIPTION

Stand erect, with feet shoulder width apart, knees slightly bent. Extend both arms in front of you, and grasp an imaginary barbell. Begin to roll it towards you, feeling the tension in your wrists and hands. After rolling the barbell forward, reverse your direction. Keep elbows and shoulders stationary during the exercise.

NUMBER OF REPETITIONS

Beginner: 5 repetitions
Intermediate: 10 repetitions
Advanced: 15 repetitions

COUNT

This exercise should be done to a count of 6.

1,2,3. forwards roll
4,5,6. backwards roll

VARIATIONS

Hold the imaginary barbell closer to your body by tucking and bending elbows in when you perform the rolling movements.

EFFECTS

This strengthens the powerful muscles around the wrist in the lower forearm. It also increases the flexibility of the fingers.

MARTIAL ARTS BENEFITS

The hand and wrist muscles are used in all grappling techniques. Strong hand and forearm muscles are also important in delivering effective blows.

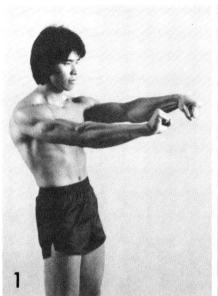
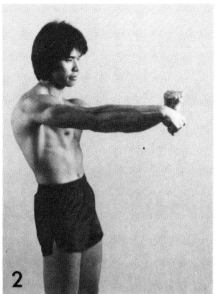
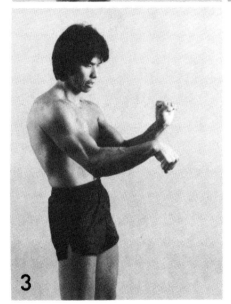

1. Standing erect, extend both arms in front of you, and grasp an imaginary barbell.
2. Begin rolling the barbell towards you, feeling the tension in your wrist and hands.
3. After rolling the barbell forward, reverse your direction. Keep elbows and shoulders stationary throughout the exercise.

WRIST ROLL

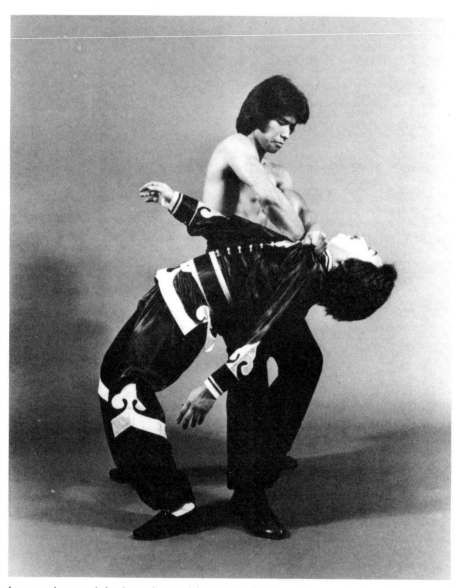

Increased strength in the wrists and forearms allows you to execute simultaneous grabs and blows with maximum effect.

LEG CONDITIONERS

These exercises concentrate on the four major muscle groups in the legs: the front of the thigh (quadriceps); the hamstrings on the back of the thigh (biceps femoris); the hip muscles; and the calves. Strong, flexible ankles are also developed through these exercises.

LEG EXTENSION

DESCRIPTION

Stand erect, with feet at shoulder width apart, knees slightly bent. Turn your left foot at a 45 degree angle, shifting all weight onto the left leg. Bend your right knee as you bring up your right leg as high as possible, supporting the upper leg with your hand. Extend the lower leg until it is in a straight line with the upper leg. The knees may be locked. The thigh muscle should be relaxed and the calf muscles tensed in this position. Your toes should be pointed straight up, towards the ceiling. (For variation, you may point the foot in line with the legs.) Slowly relax the calf and bend the knee to let the lower leg swing freely.

NUMBER OF REPETITIONS

Beginner: 5 repetitions
Intermediate: 10 repetitions
Advanced: 15 repetitions

COUNT

This exercise should be done to a count of 5.

1-4. raising the calf up
5. releasing the calf

EFFECTS

This is an intensive conditioner of the calf and hamstring muscles. As you do the upward movement, you should feel tension down the entire length of the leg. The stretch enhances flexibility, while the tension in the calf indicates the build up of muscles.

MARTIAL ARTS BENEFITS

This strengthens the vital muscles used for kicking. Your power should be vastly improved on instep or heel kicks.

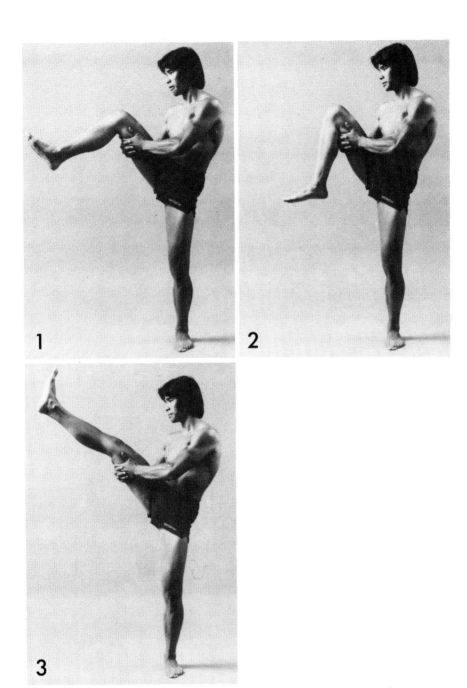

1. Bring your right leg up as high as possible, supporting the upper leg with your hand.
2. Begin extending the lower leg until...
3. It is in a straight line with the upper leg.

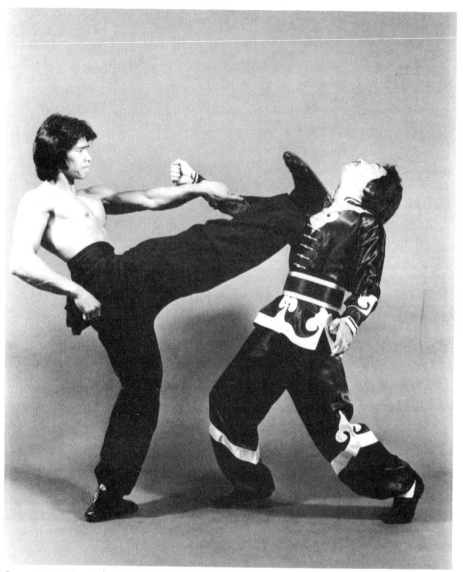

Powerful kicks through the leg's full range of motion require the flexibility and strength developed by leg extension exercises.

CALF EXTENSIONS

DESCRIPTION

Stand erect, with feet shoulder width apart, knees slightly bent. Bend over to place your hands on the floor in front of your feet. Do not bend your knees, and keep your heels on the floor throughout the exercise. Put your weight on your hands, and begin walking forward. When you reach the extreme point of your stretch, pause for 3 seconds and begin walking backwards. Return to an upright position.

NUMBER OF REPETITIONS

Beginner: 3 repetitions.
Intermediate: 6 repetitions
Advanced: 9 repetitions

COUNT

This exercise should be done to a count of 6.

1,2,3. walking forward
4,5,6. walking back

EFFECTS

This exercise excells in stretching the calf muscles and loosening tight hamstrings.

MARTIAL ARTS BENEFITS

The martial artist will find this exercise improves his ability to push off from the calves for forward and backwards movement. This will provide a more explosive and powerful forward thrust and retreat. The development of leg strength enhances all aspects of mobility and footwork needed for advance and retreat.

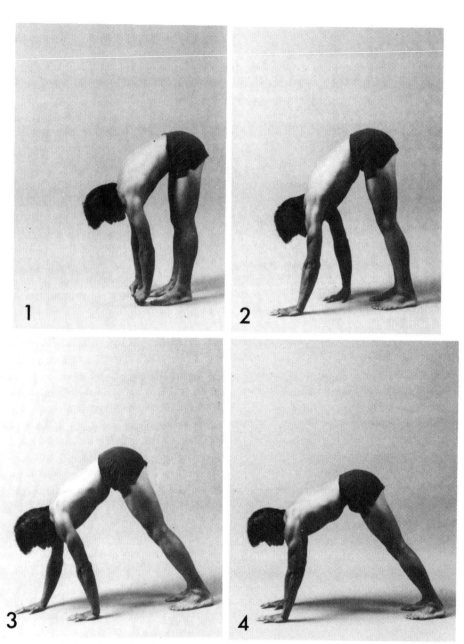

1. Bend over to place your hands on the floor in front of your feet.
2. Put your weight on your hands and begin walking forwards.
3. Continue walking forward until you reach the extreme point of your stretch.
4. Pause for three second before you begin walking backwards.

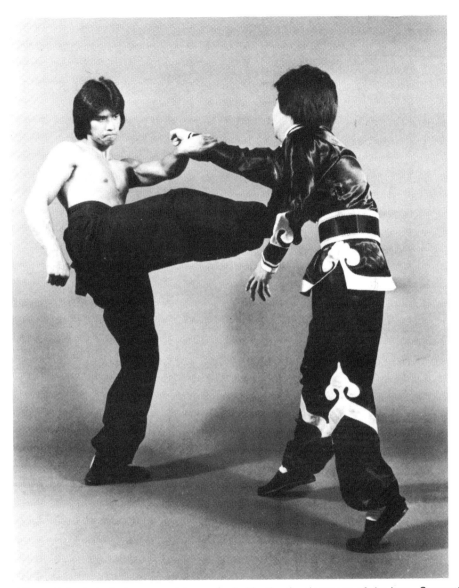

All martial arts techniques must be grounded in the development of the legs. Strength and flexibility in calf and hamstring muscles are vital in maintaining your balance. With this power base, you can generate explosive kicks without losing your foundation.

LEG PULL

DESCRIPTION

Begin in an erect stance, with feet shoulder width apart, knees slightly bent. As in the leg extension, bend your knee to bring up the left leg. Hold the front of your knee with your left hand. Hold the instep of the left foot with the right hand. Pull the knee and foot tightly to your chest, and hold for the correct count. Release the leg and repeat with the other leg. Focus on maintaining balance and agility.

NUMBER OF REPETITIONS

Beginner: 5 repetitions
Intermediate: 10 repetitions
Advanced: 15 repetitions

COUNT

Hold the extreme position for a count of 5 or more.

EFFECTS

This is an excellent stretcher and strengthener for the quadriceps (front of thighs), calves, and ankles. The lower back, pelvic and hip muscles will also be toned.

MARTIAL ARTS BENEFITS

The balance developed by this exercise is essential for power. It will also strengthen the specific muscles used for jamming, in side kicks, and for general mobility.

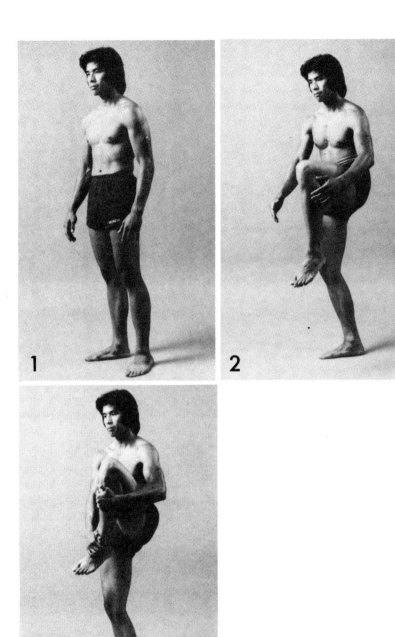

1. Begin in an erect stance, feet shoulder width apart, knees slightly bent.
2. Bend your knee to bring up the left leg.
3. Hold the front of your knee with your left hand, and the instep of the left foot with your right hand. Pull the knee and foot tightly to your chest.

LEG PULL

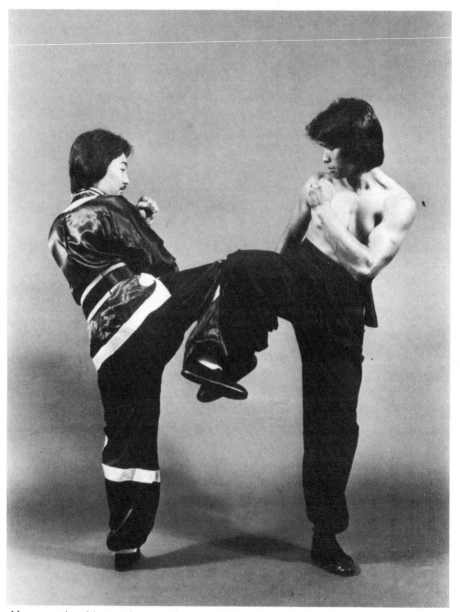

You must be able to raise your knee quickly and powerfully in order to block attempted kicks.

SQUATS

DESCRIPTION

Stand erect, with feet shoulder width apart, with your hands on your waist. Keeping your back straight and your buttocks tucked in, begin to slowly bend your knees, squatting down. Imagine that a weighted barbell has been placed across your back. Continue to lower your body, bending your knees until you are about halfway down to the ground. Make sure that your knees are not extended beyond your toes. Curl your toes as if grabbing the ground, and concentrate on hollowing your arches. Then, just as slowly, begin rising to a standing position, until you are back in the starting position.

NUMBER OF REPETITIONS

Beginner: 8 repetitions
Intermediate: 16 repetitions
Advanced: 24 repetitions

COUNT

This exercise should be done to a count of 4.

1,2. downward movement
3,4. upward movement

EFFECTS

This exercise strengthens the hamstrings, quadriceps and calf muscles, and is an intensive conditioner for all the muscles in the feet. It also firms and tightens the pelvic area and buttocks. Because the arms are not used for balance, it is excellent practice for developing balance and stability.

MARTIAL ARTS BENEFITS

Balance is the foundation of the martial arts. You must have a solid foundation, by being rooted to the floor, to develop balance and agility. This solid foundation, which allows you a base for attack or defense, requires exceptionally strong leg muscles. Strong legs are essential for exploding kicks through your opponent.

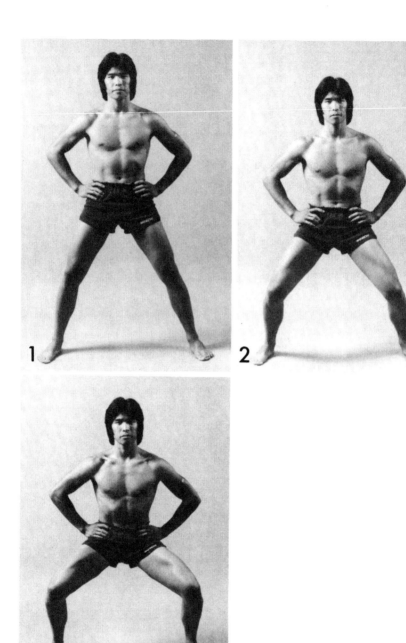

1. Stand erect, feet shoulder width apart, with hands on your waist.
2. Keeping your back straight and your buttocks tucked in, begin to bend your knees slowly, squatting down.
3. Continue to lower your body, bending your knees until you are about halfway down to the ground. Curl your toes as if grabbing the ground, and hollow your arches.

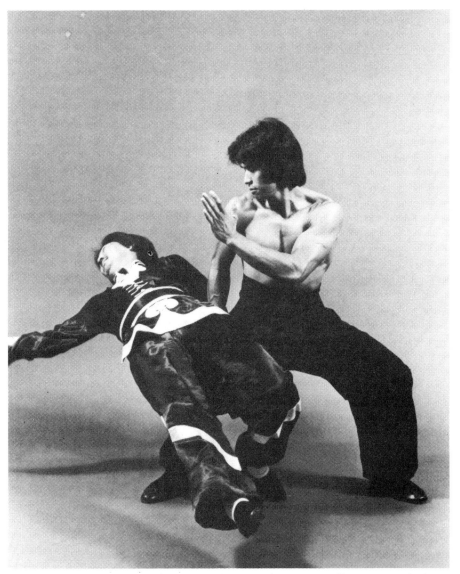

With a solid foundation rooting you to the ground you can easily execute takedowns without upsetting your balance.

HORSES

DESCRIPTION

Begin in a bow and arrow stance. Very slowly, begin to shift weight to your lead leg. When you have shifted all the weight you can without losing your balance, just as slowly begin shifting your weight back to your rear leg. Continue this shifting movement. Then change your stance to make the other leg become the lead leg.

After you shift your weight, you should be able to lift the unweighted foot without losing your balance. However, even in your extreme position, you should not have your knee extending beyond your toes.

As you do this exercise, be conscious of tilting your pelvis to tuck your buttocks under your body. Remember to maintain your feet below the body at all times.

NUMBER OF REPETITIONS

Beginner: 5 repetitions
Intermediate: 10 repetitions
Advanced: 15 repetitions

COUNT

This exercise should be done to a count of 3. Advanced students may do the exercise faster.

EFFECTS

This is an excellent exercise for strengthening all of the leg muscles, including the muscles of the ankle. It will also strengthen the pelvic area and the buttock muscles.

MARTIAL ARTS BENEFITS

This shifting stance helps the martial artist practice advancing to deliver blows and retreating from blows without changing ground. This is a very effective technique in sparring by slipping and countering the blows.

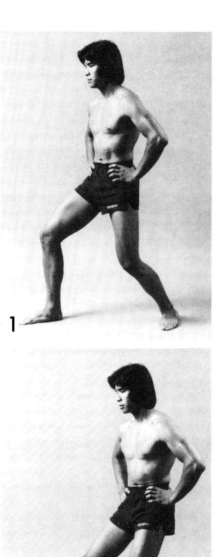

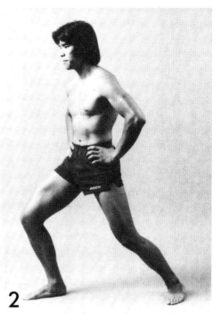

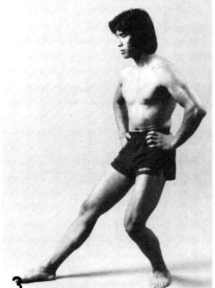

1. Assume a bow and arrow stance.
2. Begin shifting weight to your lead leg.
3. When you have shifted all the weight you can, begin shifting your weight back to your rear leg.

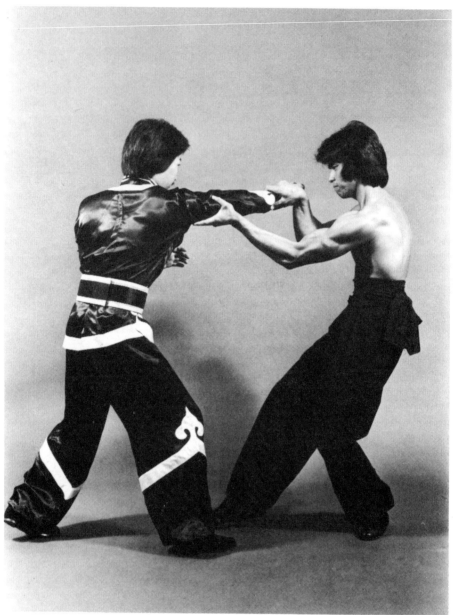

Shift your weight while keeping a powerful, rooted stance to bring your opponent first off balance, then down.

MOVING THE HORSE (TAI CHI WALK)

DESCRIPTION

This is a moving exercise, so be sure to allow plenty of room before you begin to practice it.

Begin in a bow and arrow stance with the right foot as the lead foot. Shift your weight to the left rear foot. Then turn the lead foot to the right at a 45 degree angle. Slowly transfer your weight onto the right lead foot. The left foot follows the right heel, then turns out to the left at a 45 degree angle. Now slowly transfer your weight onto the left foot. Repeat the motion by moving your right leg up to the lead leg, and stepping out at a 45 degree angle to the right.

Throughout the exercise, do not bob your head up and down, but keep it at one level. Turn your waist as you shift your weight. Your knees must always be over your toes when transferring your weight to the lead foot.

NUMBER OF REPETITIONS

Beginner: 3 repetitions
Intermediate: 6 repetitions
Advanced: 9 repetitions

COUNT

This exercise should be done to a count of 2.

1. right leg takes its step
2. left leg takes its step

EFFECTS

This exercise strengthens all the leg muscles, and is especially helpful for the flexibility and strength of the ankles. The turning motion of the waist increases the loosening of the waist and pelvic areas.

MARTIAL ARTS BENEFITS

This exercise is excellent training in smoothly transferring weight. By moving with grace, balance, and agility you will be able to avoid telegraphing your movements. This is a vital element in martial arts success.

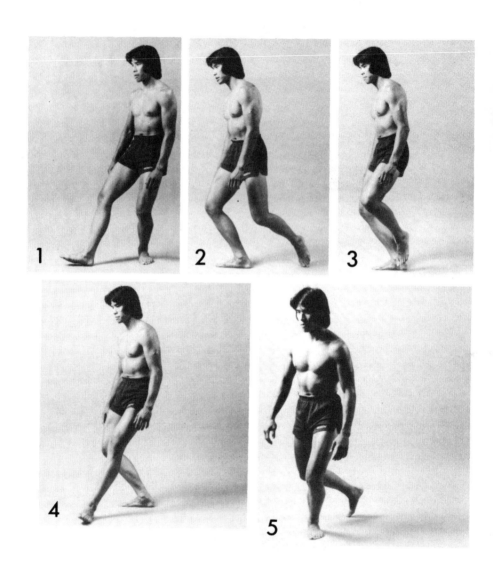

1. From a bow and arrow stance, shift your weight to the left rear foot and turn the lead right foot to the right at a 45 degree angle.
2. Slowly transfer your weight to the right lead foot.
3. Move the left foot to the right heel...
4. And then out at a 45 degree angle.
5. Slowly transfer your weight onto the left lead foot.

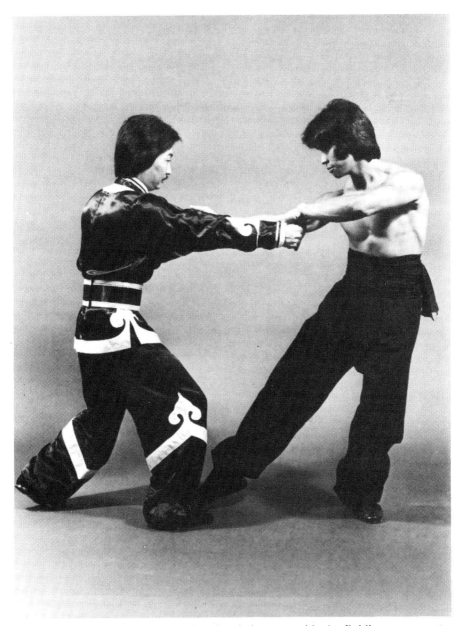

Highly developed leg muscles and perfect balance provide the fluidity necessary to attack without telegraphing your movements.

NECK CONDITIONER

Neck muscles are usually the most neglected muscles exercised, even though they protect the most vulnerable areas of the human body.

DESCRIPTION

Begin in an erect stance. Place the fingers of both hands on your forehead, and use your fingers to push your head back. At the same time, resist this backwards pressure. When your head has been pushed all the way back, begin bending your head forward. At the same time, resist the movement with the fingers of your hands. Repeat this process on both sides of your head and from different angles on your head.

NUMBER OF REPETITIONS

Beginner: 3 repetitions in each angle
Intermediate: 6 repetitions in each angle
Advanced: 9 repetitions in each angle

COUNT

This exercise should be done slowly and evenly, using a count of two.

EFFECTS

Because the exercise can be performed from every angle, it evenly and progressively strengthens all of your neck muscles. These neck muscles are not only important in making head movements smooth and flexible, but they also protect your vulnerable spinal cord and windpipe. Since important centers of the nervous, circulatory, and respiratory systems are all located in the neck, strong neck muscles are vital for your health and protection.

MARTIAL ARTS BENEFITS

The ability to move your head quickly to every angle and position will be invaluable in sparring situations. If your opponent aims a blow to your head, you can move your head the precise amount of distance necessary to avoid it. If a blow lands, your increased flexibility will better enable you to withstand it. This muscular development also enhances your speed and control.

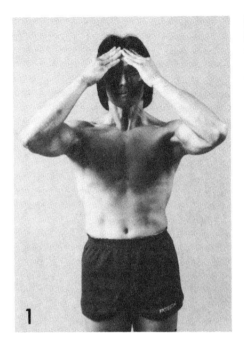 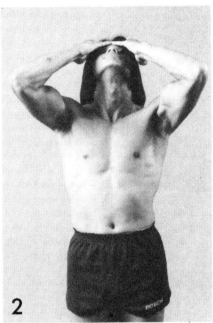

1. Stand erect with feet at shoulder width apart. Place your fingers on your forehead and begin pushing your head back.

2. Push your head all the way back, resisting the backwards pressure. Then begin pushing your head foreward.

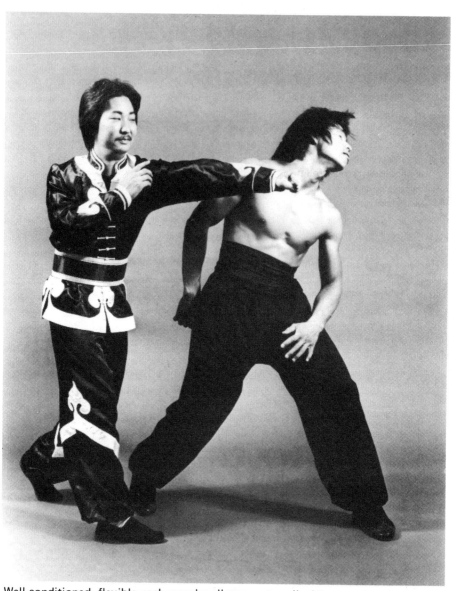

Well-conditioned, flexible neck muscles allow you to roll with a punch and avoid absorbing the full impact of the opponent's blow.

Training

You should set up a training schedule to suit your needs before you begin the dynamic strength exercises. The training schedules which follow are sample programs for beginning, intermediate and advanced students. They can be used by any individual who wants to improve general strength and flexibility. As you progress, you should gradually increase both the amount of tension you use in practicing and the number of repetitions of each exercise. Devise your own variations on the basic schedule, depending on the amount of time you will be able to spend and the parts of the body you want to emphasize.

You should work out (following your chosen program) every other day. On the off days, you may wish to practice the basic warm-up exercises. However, since strength and muscle mass increase while the body is resting, it is best not to train two days in a row.

Put aside a set time each day in which to exercise. This will accustom your body to working out at that time each day. Be sure to schedule your work out at least one hour before or after eating. If you eat before the session, you may feel sluggish or get stomach cramps while exercising. You will also not want to eat until at least an hour after exercise since vigorous workouts inhibit the appetite.

You can perform these exercises anywhere, as no equipment is necessary. However, it is best to train in some spacious, well-ventilated area where you can be alone. This will enhance your concentration, which is vital for dynamic strength exercises. As mentioned earlier, a full-length mirror will help you make sure you are practicing the exercises correctly.

After doing any new set of exercises, you will probably experience some soreness or muscle stiffness. You should be pleased, as this is a sign that your muscles are increasing in strength. Massage and hot baths are helpful to relieve the pain.

Do not continue any exercise if you feel pain or undue stress. Although it is unlikely you will hurt yourself if you practice the exercises correctly, jerky movements can strain or tear muscle fibers and should be avoided.

In evaluating your progress, you will notice that some improvements will be immediate, such as better body posture. By taking inventory of your physique in a mirror, you will immediately make adjustments to correct how erect you hold your body, the position of your shoulders, etc. Other results will take a greater length of time to become apparent. As in any exercise program, it takes time to reach your goals. However, after a few weeks, you should begin to notice some gains. You will be able to monitor your progress in many ways. By checking your actions in a mirror, you'll be able to see noticeable improvements in your movements. You will be able to feel the increase in muscle mass and experience the sensation of power in increased strength. You will also be aware that your breathing becomes easier, less strenuous and more measured as you gain proficiency in the dynamic strength exercises.

BEGINNERS' PROGRAM

Use the number of repetitions indicated for the beginning student.

Warm-Up Exercises:

1. Mental Preparation—The Three A's: Be Awake; Aware; and Alertly Relaxed
2. Neck Rotation
3. Upper Torso Rotation
4. Shoulder Rotations
5. Hip Rotation
6. Knee Rotation
7. Knee Bends

Dynamic Strength Exercises

1. Whisking Arms
2. Torso Twisting
3. Finger Exercise
4. Crane Hand
5. Leg Pull
6. Squats
7. Horses

INTERMEDIATE PROGRAM

The same as for the beginner, except you should graduate to the number of repetitions indicted for the intermediate students and add a few additional warm-up and dynamic strength exercises.

Additional Warm-Up Exercises:

1. Backwards arm swing
2. Push-ups
3. Leg raises

Additional Dynamic Tension Exercises:

1. Vertical Palm Press
2. Prayer Press
3. Curls
4. French Curls
5. Moving the Horse
6. Neck Exercise

ADVANCED PROGRAM

Same as for the beginner and intermediate, except you should graduate to the number of repetitions indicted for the advanced student. At this level, dynamic strength can supplement your regular work out routine or be a complete one in itself. The advanced student should try all the exercises, picking out the ones that best fit his needs and wants. Continue practicing the exercises that you find are comfortable, exciting, and which best complement your regular routine. The Wrist Roll, Moving the Horse, Crossing Hands, Finger Exercise, Horses, and Pulleys are particularly demanding exercises if done correctly. Concentration and awareness are the main ingredients for achievement.

ABOUT THE AUTHOR

Harry Wong's life-long experiences in the martial arts and body building are the background to the development of this book. He has been involved with various martial arts for the past 33 years. Beginning with Grand Master Jimmy H. Woo, he has achieved the status of Master in San Soo Kung Fu. He is currently studying Tai Chi Chuan, Hsing Yi Chuan and Ba-Gua Zhang under Grand Master Wang, Shi Qing, the National Champion of China in Push Hands and San Shou.

Mr. Wong's martial arts training is complemented by his involvement in body building. He has studied and experimented with the use of weights, isometrics and dynamic tension in his physical development.

Mr. Wong's skills in the martial arts have led to his activity in the movie and television industry. His credits as an actor and stuntman include frequent appearances on the *Kung Fu* TV series, as well as appearances in *Ironside*, *The Quest* and *When Hell Was in Session*.